T0332489

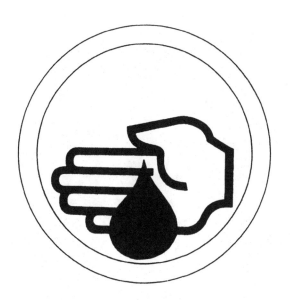

DEVELOPMENTS IN HEMATOLOGY AND IMMUNOLOGY

Volume 27

Transfusion Medicine: Fact and Fiction

Proceedings of the Sixteenth International Symposium on Blood Transfusion, Groningen 1991, organized by the Red Cross Blood Bank Groningen-Drenthe

edited by

C. Th. SMIT SIBINGA and P. C. DAS
Red Cross Blood Bank Groningen-Drenthe, The Netherlands

and

J. D. CASH
Scottish National Blood Transfusion Centre, Edinburgh, Scotland

 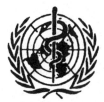

This 16th International Symposium on Blood Transfusion was conducted under the auspices of:
the International Society of Blood Transfusion (ISBT)
the World Health Organization (WHO)
the Secretary-General of the Council of Europe (Ms Catherine Lalumière)

KLUWER ACADEMIC PUBLISHERS
DORDRECHT / BOSTON / LONDON

Library of Congress Cataloging-in-Publication Data

Symposium on Blood Transfusion (16th : 1991 : Groningen, Netherlands)
    Transfusion medicine : fact and fiction : proceedings of the 16th
Anual Symposion on Blood Transfusion, Groningen 1991 / organised by
the Red Cross Blood Bank Groningen-Drente ; edited by C. Th. Smit
Sibinga and P.C. Das, and J.D. Cash.
        p.   cm. -- (Developments in hematology and immunology ; v. 27)
    Includes index.
    ISBN 0-7923-1732-7 (HB : alk. paper)
    1. Blood--Transfusion--Congresses.   I. Smit Sibinga, C. Th.
II. Das, P. C.   III. Cash, J. D. (John David)   IV. Stichting Rode
Kruis Bloedbank Groningen/Drente.   V. Title.   VI. Series.
    [DNLM: 1. Blood Banks--organization & administration--congresses.
2. Blood Transfusion--congresses.   W1 DE997VZK v.27 / WB 356 S989g
1991]
RM171S93 1991
362.1'784--dc20
DNLM/DLC
for Library of Congress   92-12547

ISBN 0-7923-1732-7

Published by Kluwer Academic Publishers,
P.O. Box 17, 3300 AA Dordrecht, The Netherlands.

Kluwer Academic Publishers incorporates
the publishing programmes of
D. Reidel, Martinus Nijhoff, Dr W. Junk and MTP Press.

Sold and distributed in the U.S.A. and Canada
by Kluwer Academic Publishers,
101 Philip Drive, Norwell, MA 02061, U.S.A.

In all other countries, sold and distributed
by Kluwer Academic Publishers Group,
P.O. Box 322, 3300 AH Dordrecht, The Netherlands.

Printed on acid-free paper

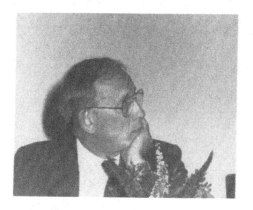 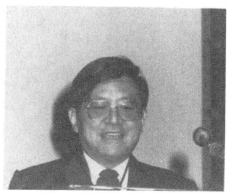

Prof. J. D. Cash,
chairman

Dr. Hu Ching-Li,
assistant director-general WHO

Facts and Fictions: They are not always easy to distinguish.

from: Monsignor Quixote
      Graham Greene, 1984

Transfusion Medicine deals with that part of the health care system, which undertakes the approprate provision and use of human blood resources.

If we make the working assumption that Transfusion Practice is that collective activity which links the blood donor with the patient, than it follows that Transfusion Medicine occupies those areas in which it is deemed important or even essential that a medical practitioner contributes to this bridging process.

WHO/GBSI 1991

Baxter

Acknowledgement

This publication has been made possible through the support of Baxter, which is gratefully acknowledged.

CONTENTS

MODERATORS AND SPEAKERS

Moderators

J.D. Cash (chairman)	– Scottish National Blood Transfusion Centre Edinburgh, UK
W.G. van Aken	– Central Laboratory for the Blood Transfusion Amsterdam, NL
P.C. Das	– Red Cross Blood Bank Groningen-Drenthe Groningen, NL
C. Dudok de Wit	– Blood Transfusion Council Amsterdam, NL
B. Habibi	– National Blood Transfusion Centre Paris, F
U. Rossi	– Department of Haematology and Blood Transfusion Centre Legnano, I
C.Th. Smit Sibinga	– Red Cross Blood Bank Groningen-Drenthe Groningen, NL
T.F. Zuck	– Paul Hoxworth Blood Center Cincinnati, OH, USA

Speakers

R.W. Beal	– League of Red Cross and Red Crescent Societies Geneva, CH
H.J.ten Duis	– University Hospital Groningen Groningen, NL
J.S. Epstein	– Department of Health & Human Services, Food and Drug Administration Bethesda, MD, USA
J.D. Evans	– Trent Regional Health Authorities Sheffield, UK

J.K.M. Gevers	– University of Amsterdam Amsterdam, NL
W.N. Gibbs	– World Health Organization Geneva, CH
D. Goldfinger	– Cedars-Sinai Medical Center Los Angeles, CA, USA
C.F. Högman	– University Hospital Blood Bank Uppsala, S
H.G. Klein	– National Institutes of Health Bethesda, MD, USA
A.P.M. Los	– Red Cross Blood Bank Groningen-Drenthe Groningen, NL
J.E. Menitove	– Paul Hoxworth Blood Centre Cincinnati, OH, USA
B.T. Teague	– Gulf Coast Regional Blood Center Houston, TX, USA
S.J. Urbaniak	– Aberdeen and North-East of Scotland Blood Transfusion Service Aberdeen, UK
W. Wagstaff	–National Blood Transfusion Service Sheffield, UK

Prepared Discussants

| G. Matthes | – Institute of Transfusiology, Medical School (Charité)
Berlin, D |
| Y. Piquet | – Regional Blood Transfusion Service
Bordeaux, F |

OPENING ADDRESS AND INTRODUCTORY LECTURE: THE GLOBAL BLOOD SAFETY INITIATIVE

Dr. Hu Ching-Li
Assistant Director-General World Health Organization

On behalf of the World Health Organization (WHO) it is my pleasure to open this Symposium, and thus demonstrate the importance which the Organization places on blood safety.

To use a Chinese proverb, I want to throw the stone in order to attract the jade or the goat. You are the experts and I throw the stone to test where we have to go because of this jade. WHO is coming here to listen to you, the experts, to your advice, to your opinions. This will bring WHO in a better position to serve the countries, particularly those in the developing world.

For more than two decades the World Health Organization, in collaboration with governments and other organizations, has promoted the establishment and development of blood transfusion services.

Resolution WHA28.72 adopted by the Twenty-eighth World Health Assembly in 1975 urged Member States to "promote the development of national blood services based on voluntary non-remunerated donation of blood", and requested the Director-General to increase assistance to Member States for this purpose, "when appropriate in collaboration with the League of Red Cross Societies" [1].

During its seventy-nineth session in 1987 the Executive Board adopted resolution EB79.R1, reiterating the Board's support for WHA28.72. The director-General was requested to support Member States in developing national policies for blood and blood products and using them rationally. It also requested him to "update and make available to Member States ... valid information related to blood, blood products and blood substitutes, and on appropriate and cost-effective ways of organizing blood transfusion services" [2].

The technical programmes within WHO responsible for carrying out these mandates have worked in close collaboration with organizations such as the League of Red Cross and Red Crescent Societies (LRCS), the International Society of Blood Transfusion (ISBT), the World Federation of Hemophilia (WFH) and the International Federation of Blood Donor Organizations (FIODS).

This work has embraced all aspects of what is now known as Transfusion Medicine:
1. blood donor recruitment and retention;
2. collection, processing and storage of blood and blood products; and
3. appropriate use of blood.

This has always been done in the context of trying to improve the organization of the blood transfusion services, including quality assurance. Activities have included recruitment of experts for assessing needs, preparing project proposals and serving as project officers in establishing or improving blood transfusion services; training, including the organization of courses and workshops and the preparation of guidelines and training materials; and supply of equipment, reagents and other material.

More recently, the AIDS pandemic has increased awareness of the need for ensuring the safety of blood and blood products. It is estimated that globally about 10% of all AIDS cases are attributable to transfusion of blood and blood products. However, the proportion varies considerably between countries – from considerably less than 1% in developed countries to nearly 20% in some developing countries. In some groups within the latter (e.g., children) the proportion of AIDS cases attributed to transfused blood or blood products is as high as 30% or 40%. Moreover, HIV transmission by blood transfusion in about 95% efficient, where the effectiveness of HIV transmission by sexual activities is around 25%.

In 1988 WHO's Global Programme on AIDS (GPA), in collaboration with the unit of Health Laboratory Technology and Blood Safety (LBS), LRCS, ISBT and the United Nations Development Programme (UNDP) launched the Global Blood Safety Initiative (GBSI) with the main objective of ensuring safe, adequate supplies of blood and blood products, which are effective and accessible at reasonable costs to those who need them. It was felt that this could best be achieved through the development of integrated blood transfusion services [3].

Thus, although the objective has not changed, the launch of the GBSI marks an intensification of the effort to achieve it and an attempt to enhance collaboration between the governments, organizations, institutions and individuals involved. It is pertinent to examine the global status of blood transfusion services and to try to define the goals more precisely. I shall do this briefly, reviewing in turn the organization of the blood transfusion services:
1. blood donor recruitment;
2. collection and processing (particularly screening for infectious agents); and
3. appropriate use of blood.

A recently recommended classification of countries is used as the basis for this review:

a. developed market-economy countries or areas (DMCs)   27
b. Eastern European countries (EUCs)   8
c. developing countries or areas (DGCs)   106
d. least developed countries or areas (LDCs)   45

The 27 developed market-economy countries (DMCs) comprise Australia, Canada, Japan, New Zealand, South Africa and USA, and most of the countries in WHO's European Region which includes Israël. The estimated amount per capita spent on health (Figure 1) is highest among this group (median US$672 per year).

The 106 developing countries or areas (DGCs) are distributed in all WHO Regions, but there are only two in the European Region. The estimated amount spent on health is much lower than that for the developed countries (median US$63 per capita per year).

Most of the 45 least developed countries or areas (LDCs) are in the African and South-East Asia Regions. There are only four in the Western Pacific Region, one in the American Region and none in the European Region. The median of the estimated amount spent on health in this group per year per capita is US$10.

The corresponding figure for Eastern European countries (EUCs) is US$280.

Global status of blood transfusion services

Organization of transfusion services

Uncoordinated hospital-based transfusion services are inefficient and increase the risk of unsafe practices. 60% of the blood transfusion services in develo-

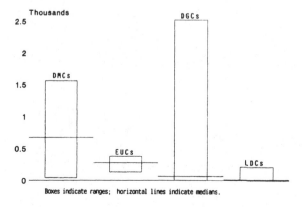

Boxes indicate ranges; horizontal lines indicate medians.

Figure 1. Estimated amounts spent on health (US$ per capita per year).

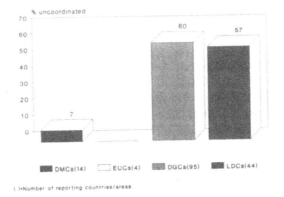

Figure 2. Uncoordinated hospital-based BTS.

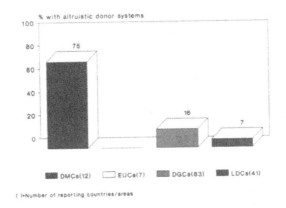

Figure 3. Altruistic blood donor systems.

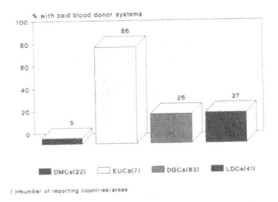

Figure 4. Paid blood donor systems.

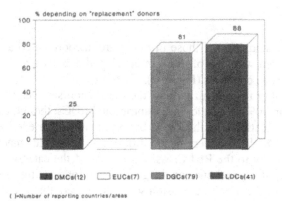

Figure 5. Dependence on "replacement" donors.

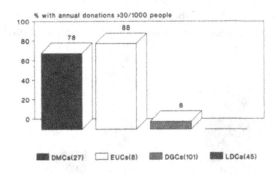

Figure 6. Annual blood donations; related to population.

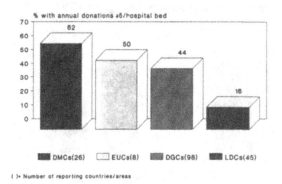

Figure 7. Annual blood donations; related to hospital beds.

ping countries and 57% of those in LDCs are uncoordinated and hospital-based, compared with 7% of those in developed countries and none in the Eastern European countries (Figure 2).

Responsibility for organization of the transfusion services rests with the government in 90% of developing countries and LDCs, though this is some-times in collaboration with the Red Cross, another NGO or even with private enterprise. 39% of the governments of developed countries have delegated this responsibility to the Red Cross. Regardless of the category of country there is nearly always reliance on the government for meeting capital and re-current costs of the blood transfusion services. Indeed, this is a dilemma for developing countries and LDCs, and it is not surprising that the Red Cross and/or funding agencies provide additional aid to 33% and 54% of these coun-tries, respectively.

Donor recruitment and selection

The quality of the blood and blood products transfused is determined to a large extent by the quality of the blood supply. Several studies have shown that voluntary non-remunerated blood donors present the smallest risk of

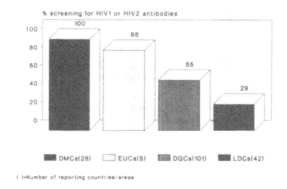

Figure 8. Markers for infectious agents; HIV1/HIV2.

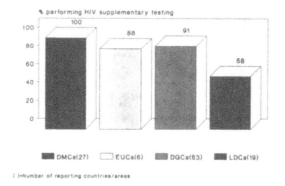

Figure 9. Markers for infectious agents; HIV supplementary testing.

transmitting infectious agents and that this risk increases considerably among paid donors. There are also indications that the risk is high among replacement or family donors in some countries. This is because many of the donors in this category in some countries are in fact paid blood donors.

75% of developed countries depend entirely on non-remunerated blood donors whereas this applies only to 16% of the developing countries and 7% of LDCs (Figure 3).

There are paid blood donors in 5% of developed countries, 26% of developing countries and 27% of LDCs, and 86% of the Eastern European countries (Figure 4). More than 80% of the developing countries and LDCs depend partially or entirely on replacement donors compared with 25% of developed countries (Figure 5).

There are indications, also, that the amount of blood collected in developing countries and LDCs is insufficient to meet their needs.

There are 30 or more donations per 1000 of the population in 78% of the developed and 88% of Eastern European countries, but only in 8% of developing countries and in none of the LDCs (Figure 6).

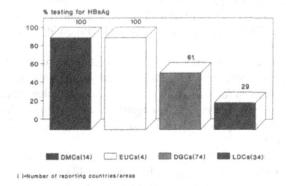

Figure 10. Markers for infectious agents; HBsAg.

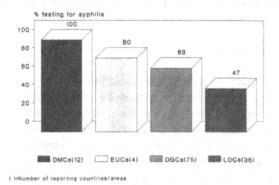

Figure 11. Markers for infectious agents; syphilis.

Corresponding figures for five or more donations per hospital bed are: 62% of developed countries, 50% of the Eastern European countries, 44% of developing countries and 16% of LDCs (Figure 7).

Unfortunately, there is insufficient information on the availability of systems for blood donor selection and self-exclusion, on donor record systems and on facilities to trace donors and recipients. However, there are indications that less than half of the developing countries and LDCs have these systems established.

Processing of blood

Increased attention has been focused recently on the ability of countries to screen for markers of infectious agents transmissible by blood. HIV seropositivity is demonstrable in up to 20% of blood donors in some countries, and the prevalence of hepatitis B surface antigen (HBsAg) and positive serological tests for syphilis may be as high as 35% and 12%, respectively.

In developed countries all units are tested for HIV seropositivity, HBsAg and serological tests for syphilis. All HIV seropositive units are subjected to supplementary testing. 88% of Eastern European countries, 55% of developing countries and 29% of LDCs screen all blood units collected for HIV antibodies (Figure 8).

Supplementary testing on HIV seropositive units is carried out by 91% of the developing countries, 88% of the Eastern European countries, and 58% of the LDCs which screen for HIV antibodies. This marks a clear improvement over the past two years, but is clearly still unsatisfactory (Figure 9).

Only 61% of developing countries and 29% of LDCs test all units for HBsAg (Figure 10).

On the other hand, nearly 70% of developing countries and half of the LDCs perform serological tests for syphilis (Figure 11).

Although information on blood group serological testing is inadequate for a satisfactory statistical analysis, what is available indicates that this is unsatisfactory in most developing countries and LDCs. Quality assurance is also generally unsatisfactory.

Appropriate use of blood

The sparse information available suggests that the inappropriate use of blood is widespread - in all categories of countries. This includes the transfusion of blood or blood products in situations where alternative therapy is indicated. In addition, whereas in most developed countries at least 50% of the blood collected is transfused as components, in developing countries and LDCs most of the blood is transfused without separation into its components.

Most developed countries have facilities for plasma fractionation and are therefore self-sufficient, or nearly self-sufficient, in blood products. Most developing countries must import these products but have insufficient funds to do so.

Finally the availability in developing countries and LDCs of crystalloids or colloids is usually limited, and this is one of the reasons for the inappropriate use of blood for acute hemorrhage in some countries.

Summary of global status of blood transfusion services

The blood transfusion services in most countries are poorly organized, unco-ordinated and hospital-based.

Donor motivation, recruitment and selection is inadequate, resulting in insufficient numbers of donations to meet countries' needs.

At the same time there is heavy dependence on replacement donors and, in some cases, on paid donors and therefore an increased risk of transmitting infectious agents. This is compounded by inadequate systems for donor selection and exclusion, and impaired ability to trace donors and recipients.

Facilities for processing and storing blood, including the ability to screen donations for agents transmissible by blood, are often poorly developed and inadequate.

The inappropriate use of blood and blood products is widespread.

Yet, despite the rather bleak picture painted above, blood transfusion services have been organized successfully in some developing countries. Examples are Barbados, Botswana, Costa Rica, Cuba, Democratic People's Republic of Korea, Ethiopia, French Polynesia, Hong Kong, Indonesia, Iran, Jamaica, Jordan, Lesotho, Malaysia, Namibia, Nepal, New Caledonia, Papua New Guinea, Republic of Korea, Rwanda, Singapore, Somalia, Sri Lanka and Zimbabwe. This list is by no means exhaustive. To a varying extent these countries have accomplished some or all of the following:

1. organized efficient regional or national blood transfusion services, including improved management, administration and quality assurance
2. increased the number of blood donors recruited and retained, eliminating dependence on paid donors (where this may have existed previously) and, in some cases, progressing to fully voluntary non-remunerated blood donor systems
3. introduced and maintained procedures for collection, processing and storage of blood which have improved the safety of blood transfusion
4. set up procedures for appropriate use of blood and blood products
5. some of these countries are LDCs, demonstrating that even countries in this category may successfully undertake the development of efficient blood transfusion services.

These examples teach important lessons in the approach to the development of such projects. These countries have in common:
- strong government support and commitment
- strong professional leadership
- long-term sympathetic help of an external funding agency
- the necessary basic infrastructure

Role of WHO

As has been mentioned previously, the organizations involved in launching the GBSI believe that its main objective can best be achieved through the development of integrated blood transfusion services. Accordingly the GBSI Secretariat has set as a target the development of coordinated blood transfusion services in at least 70% of the countries in each WHO Region by 1995. There are four main strategies followed by WHO and its partners in GBSI Secretariat to improve blood transfusion services, taking into account the very wide variation in their state of development in different countries.

1. To facilitate the development and implementation of country projects intended for those countries in which there has been little or no development of blood transfusion services. Priority is given to those with identified needs, strong government support, professional leadership and the necessary basic infrastructure. In collaboration with its partners the GBSI has already identified such countries, has helped in assessment of needs and preparation of project proposals, and has helped or is helping to identify sources of funding. Once this stage is reached the project can proceed by direct contact between the donor and the recipient of aid. Because of the small size of the GBSI Secretariat a target of ten such projects has been set for implementation by 1995.

2. To facilitate correction of deficiencies in those countries in which there has been some development of the blood transfusion service. As already indicated during the outline of the global status, these deficiencies may be any combination of organization; blood donor recruitment; collection, processing and storage of blood or blood products; or appropriate use of blood or blood products. GBSI's activities to correct deficiencies have include 16 training courses for more than 300 participants; preparation of 14 guidelines and recommendations; and assistance in organizing and participation in five Regional Blood Safety workshops. The latter bring together decision makers in countries in the WHO Region during which discussions on adaptation of the GBSI guidelines and recommendations, and methods for resolving problems are discussed. This approach has produced tangible progress in the Western Pacific, South-East Asia and Eastern Mediterranean Regions.

There is not sufficient time available to list all of the targets related to the strategies for correcting deficiencies, and I shall mention only a few, related to blood donor recruitment, projected by the GBSI Secretariat. They hope that, by 1995, it will be possible for more than 70% of the countries in each WHO Region to have at least one trained blood donor recruitment officer; and for less than 5% of the countries in each WHO Region to have paid blood donor systems. They also hope that the decline in dependence on paid blood donors will be accompanied by a decline in dependence on replacement donors. They have therefore set a target for 1995 for most of the donations in at least half of the countries in each WHO Region to be obtained from voluntary non-remunerated donors.

3.   The GBSI's third strategy is research and development. This involves the provision of seeding funds from the GBSI to start small studies intended to provide information which will help countries to develop their blood policy and the preparation of proposals for more substantial funding. Seeding funds have been provided for eight studies, including three on the prevalence of transmissible infectious agents. Five development projects have been identified for implementation, including three on small-scale preparation of virus-free blood products.

4.   The fourth strategy is monitoring and evaluation. WHO is in a unique position to provide a global perspective on the development of blood transfusion services. Indeed, most of the data presented previously have been derived from the GBSI database, which includes information supplied by WHO's partners in this Initiative - notably the LRCS. Monitoring indicators and evaluation criteria have been drawn up, and the update information obtained periodically from the database will be used appropriately not only for assessing GBSI activities in relation to its targets, but also for measuring the progress made in developing blood transfusion services globally.

Most of the targets outlined are ambitious but achievable, given the availability of adequate resources.

   The GBSI has been fortunate in having the help of several experts concerned with the development of blood transfusion services, and has currently a database of more than 200 such individuals. However, what is now needed more than ever is the necessary funding to move forward more rapidly.

   On behalf of the World Health Organization I should like to express our sincere thanks to the organizers of this 16th International Symposium on Blood Transfusion for inviting me to address you at this opening session. I am very pleased to have this contact with you all, and I take this opportunity to urge all NGOs, governments and international agencies to give technical and financial support to the GBSI programme. I should emphasize that your support of the GBSI programme will enable us to improve rapidly the situation in the developing and the least developed countries, to achieve the target set by GBSI, and to attain our goal of Health of All.

References
1. World Health Assembly. Resolution WHA28.72, Utilization and supply of human blood products. Geneva 1975.
2. World Health Organization. EB79/1987/REC/1. Geneva 1987.
3. World Health Organization. WHO/GPA.DIR/88.9, Report of the Global Blood Safety Initiative meeting. Geneva 1988.

I. PROFESSIONAL ASPECTS

TRANSFUSION MEDICINE:
CONCEPT AND INTERDISCIPLINARY ASPECTS

B. Habibi

Transfusion medicine may be defined as the art of appropriate *provision* and *use* of human blood resources and related services.

The provision has evolved through three ages

A spectacular *childhood* overlapping the first World War. This is the *"transfusion era"* in its literal perception, starting with Karl Landsteiner's discovery of ABO blood groups and linking the donor and recipient arm to arm.

An expanding *adolescence* during and after the second World War. This is the *"blood banking era"* where anticoagulant solutions and glass bottles separate donors and recipients in time and space. Red cells and plasma are dissociated to be used separately. Edwin Cohn initiates the cold ethanol fractionation of plasma into albumin and gammaglobulins. Surgical operations which hitherto are unthinkable develop tremendously.

An enriching and tumultuous *maturity* since the 1960s. The *"transfusion medicine era"* were the revolutionary concept of component therapy is forged to found the basis of the modern transfusion practice, as a medical necessity, a scientific evidence, an ethical obligation towards blood donors and an economic requirement. Whole blood is separated into its components to treat each patient with the component he or she needs physiologically to the exclusion of other components which thus are not wasted and may benefit to other patients. Blood centres strive to prepare selectively red cells, platelets, granulocytes thanks to the development of closed plastic bag systems and later to cytapheresis machines. Progress in protein biochemistry and plasma fractionation lead to industrial equipment providing numerous therapeutically active plasma proteins for the management of distinct disease states.

All along this evolution voluntary blood donors have been the faithful companions of this adventure providing the source material needed to meet the ever increasing demand. This altruistic support of the community is a unique and essential characteristic of transfusion medicine. Among others, the French history provides a lively example of such support (Figure 1).

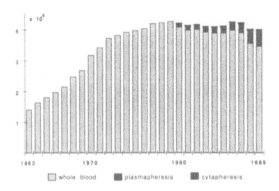

Figure 1. Blood donations in France from 1963 to 1989 showing the increasing input from the public: 1963: 1,409,000 – 1989: 4,006,000.

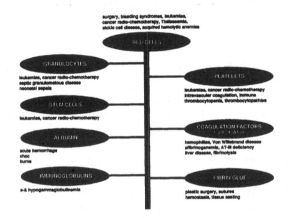

Figure 2. Main areas of human therapeutics served by blood substitution.

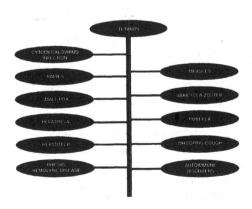

Figure 3. Main areas of passive immunotherapy by immunoglobulins.

The use covers a wide range of applications which may be divided into three areas

Replacement therapy, which aims at the compensation of potential or actual deficits in patients by giving specific and concentrated cellular blood components or plasma derivatives (Figure 2).

Passive immunotherapy through polyvalent and specific immunoglobulins, which aims at the prevention of a wide range of bacterial and viral infections as well as the treatment of autoimmune disorders (Figure 3).

Therapeutic procedures and health care services initiated in blood centres and developed in conjunction with other disciplines such as anesthesiology (autologous transfusions), neonatology (perinatal transfusion), hematology (bone marrow graft processing), oncology (ex-vivo leukocyte processing), internal medicine (hemapheresis), preventive medicine (population screening for pathologic markers, prevention of hemolytic disease of the newborn) and last but not least, immunohematologic monitoring of recipients and consultation activities.

With this brief overview in mind, one can imagine that there are sectors of human therapeutics in the development of which transfusion medicine has not played a determining role. The medical community should never take for granted or underestimate the fundamental basis of transfusion medicine's multidirectional expansion: *blood donation and blood donors*. Postage stamps commemorating voluntary blood donations express the state level recognition and the tribute governments pay or have to pay to this unique and routinely operating symbol of human solidarity.

To serve its purpose transfusion medicine has mobilized over the last half-century tremendous resources from the community, science, and industry

In developed health care systems, it has given birth to thousands of blood centres and fractionation facilities across the world, to some 30 therapeutic blood components and plasma derivatives, and as mentioned above to a wide range of technical and consultative services to patients, clinicians and the public health.

It has generated scientific concepts and applications such as component therapy, immunologic compatibility, transfusion safety, and hemapheresis each of which has opened avenues of research, scientific achievements and practical applications.

It has fostered intense intellectual activity channelled through scientific journals, newsletters, monograph series and books (Tables 1 and 2).

Table 1. Scientific journals in transfusion medicine known to the author.

- Infusionstherapie (CH)
- Journal of clinical apheresis (USA)
- Revista argentina de transfusion (ARG)
- Revista cubana de hematologia immunologia y hemoterapia (CUB)
- Revue française de transfusion et d'hémobiologie (F)
- Sangre (E)
- Transfusion (USA)
- Transfusione del sangue (I)
- Transfusion medicine (UK)
- Transfusion medicine reviews (USA)
- Transfusion science (UK)
- Vox sanguinis (CH)

It has federated workers into numerous professional and scientific associations across the world (Table 3).

Enhanced coordination is the key factor for the successful mobilization of these resources

Unlike other medical specialties the practice of transfusion medicine requires indeed a coordinated mechanism of input from several partners neither of whom can operate in isolation (Figure 4). Society's healthy donors offering the gift of source material, blood and fractionation centres as the steering entities which have to optimize collection, formulation and distribution of the gift, physicians committed to use the gift appropriately, the ultimate goal of the entire system – the patient – to acknowledge the gift, and finally the political power to coordinate partners, regulate flows, allocate resources and safeguard the donation's ethics within the community.

Transfusion medicine is unique in that it is not merely a technical exercise but a permanent endeavour to have all these partner sectors act appropriately. The key components of this endeavour are *research*, *development* and *education* to address each of the individual links of the chain with appropriate means and appropriate manpower.

One must admit however that efforts have not been evenly generated by or channelled to these partner sectors. The technical sectors of collection, preparation and fractionation have been favoured relatively whereas the extreme links of the chain, blood donation and clinical use have drained much less economic and intellectual investment in research, development and education. Furthermore, lucid eyes can readily recognize that despite the tremendous achievements outlined above, few places in the world have succeeded to attain the optimum harmony and coordination in this health care discipline. Struggle for progress has to be maintained.

Table 2. Some of the currently published information-education newsletters in transfusion medicine.

- AABB news briefs (USA)
- BBTS newsletter (UK)
- Blood bank week (USA)
- Bulletin of the Canadian society for transfusion medicine (Ca)
- Bulletin of the Netherlands society of blood transfusion (NL)
- CCBC newsletter (USA)
- Immunohematology (USA)
- Infoline – NBREP (USA)
- International blood/plasma news (USA)
- Nouvelle gazette de la transfusion (F)
- Transfusion clinique (F)
- Transfusion international (CH)
- Transfusion today (ISBT)

Table 3.

International
- International society of blood transfusion

America
- American association of blood banks
- Canadian society for transfusion medicine

Asia
- Indian society of blood transfusion and immunohaematology
- Indonesian society of hematology and blood transfusion
- Japan society of blood transfusion
- Republic of China society of blood transfusion

Europe
- British blood transfusion society
- Bulgarian society of hematology and blood transfusion
- Byelorussian republic society of hematologists and transfusionists
- Czechoslovakian society for hematology and blood transfusion
- French society of blood transfusion
- German society for transfusion medicine and immunohematology
- Italian society of immunohematology and blood transfusion
- Netherlands society of blood transfusion
- Norwegian society for immunology and transfusion medicine
- Polish society of hematology and blood transfusion
- Spanish society of blood transfusion
- Swedish society of transfusion medicine
- Yugoslavian society of hematology and blood transfusion

6

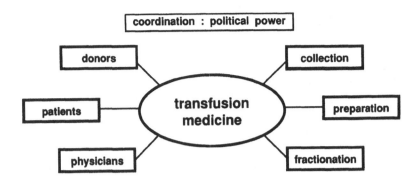

Figure 4. Operational partners in transfusion medicine.

During the last decade three factors have been instrumental in the growing perception of the critical issues to be addressed

First, the advent of AIDS and heightened recognition by physicians of the risks of other blood borne infections. Second, cost-containment pressures rising together with the necessary sophistication of therapeutic procedures and widening of the patients base. Third, increasing awareness about major inconsistencies in the use of blood resources. To explain such great disparities as those exemplified in Tables 4 and 5, in the use of blood products in countries

Table 4. France/USA disparities in the use of whole blood (WB) and red blood cell (RBC) transfusions in 1980.

	W & RBC used $\times 10^5$	Inhabitants $\times 10^6$	Use/1,000 inhabitants
France	3.3	54	61
USA	9.9	232	42

Table 5. Multiplication factors observed among developed countries in the range of consumption of some blood products.

Blood products/inhabitant	Δ range of use
RBC concentrates	× 1.8
FFP/RBC	× 2.9
Albumin kg	× 9.2
Factor VIII	× 13

with equivalent health care standards, one can hardly avoid recalling that in contrast to the provision, shaped by science and technology, the use of blood resources has long been based primarily on clinical habits and tradition.

I am convinced that with these potent catalyzers energies will be better channelled, resources better allocated and coordination better enhanced to face the challenges of the starting decade.

Challenges for the 1990s in transfusion medicine (Figure 5)

The achievement of an all voluntary blood donation system is the first major challenge to be faced in this decade by the societies, the blood transfusion professionals and the political power. The concept is based both on strong ethical principles: human solidarity, unacceptability of physical exploitation of blood donors, and on well documented medical observations of higher rate of transmissible virus carrier states (hepatitis, AIDS, etc.) among professional donors in poor socio-economic conditions. The regional and national self-sufficiency and non-remuneration of blood donations have been highlighted as a reachable goal by the European Economic Community in 1989. Donors and the Gift-relationship are the fundamental basis of transfusion medicine. It is striking to note however the relatively little social research and "low tech" means allocated to strengthen this base and to enhance the public perception and image of transfusion medicine. Needless to stress that these require in every country effective and global mobilization of the public and the public health partners.

The second major challenge is the successful management of transition to biotechnology products. Recombinant factor VIII will be on the market shortly. Growth factors have changed dramatically the use of blood cells in major clinical settings. Many blood proteins including albumin and hemoglobin have been produced by genetic engineering at the basic research level while preclinical and clinical studies are currently underway for several of these proteins such as protein C, factor VIII and anti-D immunoglobulin. The biotechnology adventure will obviously influence the blood and plasma procurement

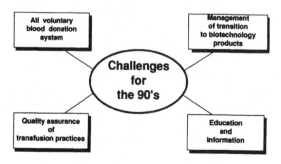

Figure 5. Challenges for the 1990s in transfusion medicine.

system if the products it generates prove to be safe, effective and inexpensive enough to complete with their natural counterparts. During this transitional period, modulating operational structures, fighting against unjustified "transfusion phobia" among patients, maintaining a still mobilized donor base, avoiding ill-advised reactions of physicians impressed by ill-founded lobbies are issues of concern to operational partners of transfusion medicine as well as the political power.

The third major challenge is the actual implementation of quality assurance programs in transfusion medicine. It is hardly provocative to maintain that fighting against human errors, negligence, hospital malpractices and ill-founded prescriptions, will prove more beneficial to patients than many of the today's or tomorrow's sophisticated laboratory screening policies.

The last major challenge is the dramatic need for education and information, one of the top priorities for the 1990s. Efforts and investments in education, information and communication should address short and medium term objectives. They should be targeted to those whose contribution is essential to the very existence of transfusion medicine, namely donors, physicians, medical students and residents, hospital partners, blood bankers and, last but not least, politicians and legislators who are responsible for setting the stage providing legal instruments to run the public health service.

To meet these challenges we need to work, to believe and to have confidence in the future.

THE PHARMACEUTICAL AND LABORATORY ASPECTS OF TRANSFUSION MEDICINE

W. Wagstaff

The pharmaceutical aspects of transfusion medicine were brought clearly into perspective in 1985 when EEC Directive number 85/374 established the rights of individuals with regard to the quality of many goods, including blood and its products. As an example of the application of this Directive, in 1987 the United Kingdom Parliament passed the Consumer Protection Act, part I of which was applicable form 1 March 1988 and introduced for the first time the concept of product liability in the field of transfusion medicine. Under this type of legislature, it is no longer necessary for an individual who has been harmed by a product to show that there had been any negligence in its production. As a consequence, most transfusion centres have now taken a structured and organized approach to quality assurance procedures, leading to the assembly of quality systems.

A typical quality system will be fully documented and will cover such aspects as management objectives, policies, organization and procedures. The objectives and policies of a typical centre will be determined by the Director in conjunction with appropriate colleagues, outlining the principles involved in the production of safe and efficacious products, the specifications of materials and services used and provided, and quality control measures taken. The specifications will cover not only the materials and reagents used in the taking and processing of blood and its components, but such other aspects as the personal health and cleanliness of donors and staff, the buildings and environmental control, and specifications of equipment including calibration and maintenance. All of these aspects may be grouped together under the common heading of Good Manufacturing Practice.

The organization of a quality system will inevitably revolve around a Quality Assurance Manager, together with all other staff responsible for functions affecting quality. The Quality Assurance Manager will be independent of production and other functions and will have appropriate authority and responsibility to make decisions and act upon the. He/she will report directly to the individual in charge of the centre, normally the Medical Director, and any conflict of views between these two individuals should be fully documented. It must be stressed however that to regard other members of staff as being "non-quality-assurance" is a totally false concept, quality assurance involves everyone. The level of responsibility which will be allowed to each number of staff, and the degree of authority necessary to discharge these responsibilities must be carefully defined. However, it should be stressed to all concerned that quality assurance is not just a laboratory function but includes everyone employed within a transfusion centre.

The key element of documentation revolves around the production of Standard Operating Procedures (SOPs). These will provide clear and documented instructions for all staff, of whatever type, on the procedures they will use in their everyday tasks. They will normally be drawn up by the most senior person routinely carrying out the procedure, and agreed with the Quality Assurance Manager. They should be readily available for consultation at any time, and should be signed by appropriate members of staff after first reading. Review and revision will take place as necessary, but this should be done at least annually. It is also necessary for a master copy of all superseded SOPs to be automatically retained as a record of procedures which once were routinely carried out in the various departments of a transfusion centre.

As an adjunct to SOPs, detailed records should be kept enabling tracing in either direction between donor and recipient, of any donation or component. These records will include at least a sessional record, a processing record, a record of inspection checks and the quality control tests, and a record of labels and/or package inserts used. It is obviously necessary for appropriate detailed records to be kept at any other link in the chain between donor and patient, for example the hospital blood bank, ward records, and the patient's medical notes.

Within the transfusion centre, a product master file will be established for each product, and will include a specification for that product, the SOPs appropriate to its generation, and the quality control procedures involved in assuring its acceptability. This master file should also include information on the type of donor or donation used in the production of the component, and a note of the suppliers of critical components used together with labelling procedures. Indeed, it is beneficial to have copies of all appropriate labels held within this product master file. The file itself should be maintained for a time determined by local legislation, for example up to 15 years in the United Kingdom.

In-house controls carried out must ensure that the processing status of any donation may be identified, including the ability to trace all components being manufactured from one donation. There should be correct inspection of the finished product and a system laid down for its authorized release. In-house protection and preservation of quality must be ensured, during storage and transport, etc., and this should be carried on to hospital level. The old view that in-house controls are confined entirely to quality control tests is no longer held, but these tests are obviously of vital importance. The test procedures themselves will be defined in accordance with the specification of the product, particularly with regard to the type of product concerned and the frequency with which the test should be carried out. The chosen tests should be subject to regular review, especially in the light of recurrent non-conformity of the product. In some instances, such non-conformity may be the fault of unsuitability of the test rather than of the product itself. Above all, it is necessary to be realistic in choice of quality control regimes, since standards set artificially high and thus resulting in a high failure rate, inevitably lead to disillusion and resentment amongst the staff preparing the component. Such resentment can have a disastrous effect on the overall application of a quality assurance program.

It is obviously necessary within such a program to identify the way in which failures will be handled. Initially, repeat tests will obviously be carried out on the same sample, and on another sample from the same batch of components to ensure that the unfavourable result is not being seen as a result of biological variation within a batch. Where non-conforming materials are identified, they must be segregated and subjected to appropriate and fully documented disposal. At the same time, procedures must be established for possible product recall and for notification of defects to institutions or individuals along the supply chain, in both directions.

The quality system itself must be subjected to a review, i.e. there must be a system of quality audit. Such a regular and systematic review is necessary to ensure the continued effectiveness of the quality system established in any centre. An external assessment at this time would be valuable if not essential. Any procedure which is revised consequent to audit must be validated before introduction as a routine in the work of the centre.

By accepting that quality assurance must represent a total scheme to ensure that any product meets specification, we go as far as we can along the road of ensuring that the pharmaceutical obligations of a transfusion service are met. We must, however, still accept the old maximum that with non-fractionated components, every donation is a batch, and under these circumstances the outcome of the transfusion may still remain somewhat unpredictable.

ROLE OF MANAGEMENT AND ADMINISTRATION IN TRANSFUSION MEDICINE

B.T. Teague

Introduction

The blood centre in Houston began operations in January of 1975 with a staff of 63 people, collections of 46,000 units of whole blood, an annual budget of $1.1 million (US), and provided services to patients in about 80 hospitals. Because of the substantial increase in patient needs in the Texas Gulf Coast area, including the world's largest medical centre (Texas Medical Center), which employs 60,000 people, we have had to grow rapidly to meet these patient needs. Today, our staff numbers over 390, we collect about 185,000 whole blood units annually, plus almost 20,000 apheresis procedures; our budget now exceeds $24 million (US); we serve 109 health care facilities, and patients in these facilities will use over 450,000 units of blood and blood components. Our greatest challenge has not been keeping up with the medical and technical aspects of this growth, but rather the administration and management aspects. Additionally, the general public, on many occasions, seems much more interested in the administrative and management aspects than the technical ones.

In my 33-year career as a blood banker, including responsibilities as a bench technologist, technical supervisor, and chief executive officer, I have been blessed to see numerous changes in our profession. In the last decade, the management and administration of blood banks has changed more than in the previous three decades combined.

Technical and medical concerns

Since the first blood bank in the United States was established in Chicago, Illinois in 1937, technological, immunological, scientific and medical concerns were appropriately given the greatest attention and resulted in major improvements in each of these areas. What tests were done, how well they were done, and the result in the patient were the focus of efforts. In the early 1970s, the need for effective administrative guidelines and their clear relationship to a successful total operation became evident. Fortunately, the American Association of Blood Banks (AABB) was a leading proponent in effecting recognition of the need and was a major contributor to its solution. The AABB has continued to offer revised Standards [1] on a periodic basis. The threat of federal legislation [2], severe criticism by the public media, local pressure and outspoken blood bankers all served as catalysts for needed changes. Administrative Guidelines [3] offer excellent ideas on public information, accounting, cooperation with other collecting groups.

Evaluation of management

The usual question is, "How do you evaluate successful management and administration performance?" In the technical and scientific arena, performance is pretty easily evaluated, based on whether or not the tests are done accurately, the number of labelling errors identified, the number of unacceptable phlebotomies performed, etc. However, it is not as easy to evaluate management and administration results.

My opinion on the criteria for evaluation is very simple! If the customers are satisfied, regulatory requirements are met, and the organization is financially sound, the management and administration have performed successfully. Without successful performance in this arena, transfusion medicine will not provide the desired result, i.e., quality service to patients.

Customer satisfaction

Customer satisfaction is the best way to gauge results in this critical area of transfusion medicine. People argue extensively on "who is the customer?" Our response to that question includes the individual volunteer donor, the donor group chairman, the corporate executives of the donor group, hospitals, hospital staff, and, probably most important, our own employees.

No matter how diligently you try to avoid mistakes in dealing with customers, mistakes are going to occur – it just happens! Management's first responsibility [4], of course, is to establish procedures which minimize the incidence of mistakes. Some organizations do a remarkably good job of this. Federal Express handles tens of thousands of shipments each working day. Some must occasionally get routed to the wrong destination, but the incidence of such errors is minuscule and complaints about Federal Express service are rarely heard.

Management's second responsibility is to establish procedures for dealing positively with such mistakes when they do occur. Few organizations do this well. If a blood centre draws 100 donors and services 99 perfectly, the one donor who has been incorrectly handled does not care that the system is 99% accurate. To retain a satisfied customer, something more is required. At a minimum, the company should acknowledge its error and express genuine regret.

Often, however, when something does go wrong – even something of a relatively minor nature – organizations respond with what is perceived as stonewalling: "No one else has had this problem"; "The problem apparently occurred as a result of your failure to give us the proper information", etc. Patronizing responses of this sort will not placate a dissatisfied customer; in fact, it will only inflame his or her negative feeling about the organization. What began as an annoying inconvenience is converted to raw animosity. The customer – more accurately the *former* customer – cannot wait to tell friends about the shabby treatment received.

The principal reason that organizations often appear arrogant in dealing with their mistakes is that routine errors tend to be committed at a fairly low corporate level. Employees responsible for the errors are less interested in customer relations than they are in covering up their own carelessness. They prefer to deny that a mistake has been made or to shift the blame for the problem to the customer.

Manager awareness

Managers are frequently unaware that internal mistakes have occurred, and they are equally in the dark with respect to the manner in which mistakes that do occur are handled. Management of every organization should work out a policy for dealing with customer dissatisfactions. The policy should be clearly communicated to employees, and here are some guidelines:
- Don't pretend to a customer that the mistake did not occur, that the mistake is not important, or that the mistake is actually the customer's fault.
  The fundamental mission of any organization is to build and nurture a core of satisfied customers. That mission is more important than the temporary embarrassment of having to confess to a mistake. If the organization errs, face up to it. Over the long pull, this will help preserve the respect and loyalty of your customers.
- Do not take the attitude that every customer who complains about a product or service is trying to pull a fast one.
  Now and again, a customer will try to take advantage, but most customers are honest. Their complaints are legitimate, or at least deserving a careful, serious investigation.
- Never deal with a customer's reported problem by responding that no one else has mentioned a similar problem. The clear message in this response is that the customer is either lying or being overly-sensitive.
- If an apology appears warranted, apologize and be gracious. People know that errors occur in the normal course of business. They are willing to accept something less than absolute perfection, but an attitude of defensive belligerence will drive customers away.

Development of these types of guidelines must be done in cooperation with the governing entity (usually the board of trustees), management of the organization, staff of the organization and, wherever possible, representatives of the customer groups.

Roles of governing body

The roles of the trustees include fiduciary (usually defined and required by law) [5], evaluation (of overall corporate performance), participatory (policy setting, not day-to-day operations), corporate resource (consultants to management and outside support), and catalyst (offering ideas and suggestions which management may not have noticed).

Roles of management

The roles of management [6], led by the chief executive officer (CEO), include productivity (only management, not nature or laws of economics or governments, makes resources productive), administration (responsibility to see that the policies approved by the board are implemented in accordance with board mandates), management (keep the board approved of operations within the corporation and select appropriate management staff to implement board policies in an effective manner), external involvement (the CEO, especially, needs to be visible in the community, so the corporation is viewed as a "good corporate citizen") and communications (the CEO is often viewed as the most credible and effective spokesperson for the organization).

Economic considerations

Economic considerations continue to be a driving force in providing services related to transfusion medicine. Only through effective management and administration will organizations be able to provide high-quality services at reasonable fees and survive in the economically-oriented climate. On more and more occasions, our customers are asking for more and more services but at reduced costs. For example, hospitals want blood and blood components tested with all available tests to insure a "safe" unit, but they do not want the service fees to go up. Most blood bankers readily admit there is no such thing as a "safe" unit of blood or blood components, in spite of all the procedures, policies, and testing involved in the recruitment, collection, testing and distribution of the unit. However, our ultimate customer, the patient, expects a 100% safe unit at a very low fee.

These are just a few of the challenges presented in transfusion medicine that relate to management and administration. Others include resource sharing, blood collected in one part of the country (or world) and shared with others in another part of the country (world). Ironically, some donors in the United States who complain that blood collected in one region was shipped to another complained even louder when more blood was not shipped from their region to the Persian Gulf during the conflict.

Summary

In summary, the technical, scientific and medical aspects of transfusion medicine continue to be critical. We all must find ways to provide a safer unit of blood and blood components. However, there must be a realization by all involved in the profession that the management and administration aspects of transfusion medicine deserve equal attention, respect and support. Why? It is very simple! Without all aspects of transfusion medicine working together for the common good – care of the patient – we will all fail.

References

1. Standards for Blood Banks and Transfusion Services, American Association of Blood Banks, 14th edition, Arlington, VA, USA, 1991.
2. Blood Assurance Act of 1979 (S.1610), Senator Richard S. Schweiker, United States Senate, Washington, DC, USA, July 31, 1979.
3. Administrative Guidelines for Blood Banks, American Association of Blood Banks, Arlington, VA, 1989.
4. "You're absolutely right: We goofed". Howard Upton, Southwest Airlines Spirit, September 1991:24.
5. Administrative Manual, Volume II, American Association of Blood Banks, Arlington, VA, USA, 1987.
6. Mueller, RK. Board management relations: Roles and values. New York: CEO Division of American Management Association, USA, 1984:17.

THE CLINICAL RESPONSIBILITIES OF TRANSFUSION MEDICINE

D. Goldfinger

In discussing the clinical responsibilities involved in the practice of transfusion medicine, I must approach this by noting that I believe there is more fiction than fact in the term "transfusion medicine" as it relates to current practices. The reasons for this are two-fold. First, the blood banker has many pressing administrative functions and is often physically removed from the patients for whom he or she has responsibility. The realities of patient care which often require direct interaction between patient and physician can be logistically difficult for blood bankers. This is particularly true when such professionals are located at donor centres remote from the hospital and certainly remote from the patient. Second, blood banking remains a highly regulated area of medical practice and much of this regulation is self-imposed. This can be seen most dramatically in reviewing the *Standards* of the American Association of Blood Banks. The practice of medicine, including transfusion medicine, is as much an art as it is a science and it must deal with the emotional as well as the scientific issues of patient care. By imposing strict rules and regulations on the manner in which a physician must practice, severe limitations are placed upon the use of ingenuity and good judgment. This is particularly a problem recently because of the medicolegal concerns facing blood bankers. As more patients are ready and willing to sue their doctors in the event of unfavourable outcomes, it becomes imperative that physicians' practices not be judged against strict rules which may not have sound scientific backing and which neglect the fact that not all practices have been proven scientifically to be both rational and safe.

The clinical responsibilities of transfusion medicine physicians include those involving both donors and patients. In the realm of donors, the management of autologous donors and of dedicated donors is of particular importance. In regard to patients, the establishment of specialized transfusion protocols for the supply of such components as leukocyte depleted components, irradiated components and CMV negative components are of special concern. In addition, the management of the acutely bleeding patient must be considered. The treatment of transfusion reactions is also a significant concern for practitioners of transfusion medicine. It is important for transfusion medicine specialists to recognize that they often have not been directly involved in the acute management of these kinds of complications for many years and are not necessarily as adept as clinical-care physicians in dealing with the kinds of complications such as shock, respiratory distress and others that often occur as part of severe reactions to blood transfusions. Yet, blood bankers often dictate what they believe to be state-of-the-art management of these reactions. Many of these dictums are decades out of date (e.g. the use of diuretics in treating acute hemolytic transfusion reactions).

This contribution will focus on a few key areas of transfusion medicine as they involve direct clinical responsibility. In this regard we must recognize our limitations and our need to keep abreast of new developments in critical care. Furthermore, transfusion medicine physicians are often too timid in dealing with severely ill patients. We do our patients a disservice if we continue to reject the care of patients who are seriously ill and focus only on those who are apparently well. While we recognize that much of our work deals with normal blood donors, the concept of transfusion medicine implies that we involve ourselves with the sick as well as the well.

Some areas in which we often have severe limitations in our clinical interactions in the realm of dealing with serious transfusion reactions will be discussed. Two issues come to mind. First, as we look at the management of acute hemolytic transfusion reactions, blood bankers have not kept abreast of significant developments in the treatment of shock and the complications of shock, namely, renal failure and pulmonary failure. In a paper published in 1977 [1], attention was called to the fact that the complications of acute hemolytic transfusion reactions were related primarily to the pathophysiology of shock and disseminated intravascular coagulation. The outcome is often renal, pulmonary and other end organ failure. Continued reliance on the use of diuretic therapy to prevent renal complications is totally out of keeping with developments of the last 20 years in the understanding of the complications of shock. Transfusion medicine specialists and the textbooks that they write continue to neglect new developments in the understanding of the pathogenesis of shock, including the importance of various vasoactive compounds that are generated in patients who are in severe shock. These are the mediators which lead to hypotension and organ failure. This knowledge should directly translate into the way we institute or recommend interventions that are capable of preventing and treating complications in patients who suffer acute hemolytic transfusion reactions. Vasoactive compounds such as histamine, bradykinin, angiotensin, prostaglandins, anaphylatoxins, tumour necrosis factor, various interleukins [2] and leukotrienes are considered to be of central importance in the development of the shock state, and interventions to alter the effects of these various mediators are crucial in treating patients and preventing serious complications. If transfusion medicine specialists feel incapable of dealing with these kinds of complex, clinical issues then they should, in fact, state this and refrain from suggesting approaches toward therapy. On the other hand, if the desire is to become involved in the management of these severely ill patients, then it is essential that we move from the dark ages of management of circulatory collapse and keep abreast of recent developments and therapeutic interventions. A good example of this is the continued failure by authors of textbook chapters on the management of these reactions to recommend the great importance of circulatory monitoring with Swan-Ganz catheters and arterial lines when dealing with these critically ill patients.

Another such example is in the management of transfusion related acute lung injury (TRALI). Many of the published recommendations of therapy regarding this disorder are clearly out of keeping with current good medical practice and the understanding of the pathogenetic mechanisms involved in this disorder. In a recent publication [3], we demonstrated that the management of this disorder with diuretic therapy to treat non-cardiogenic pulmonary edema was, in fact, potentially extremely dangerous. TRALI is a serious disorder, and results in cardiorespiratory disturbances which require the most sophisticated techniques in critical-care management. These include the placement of lines for the measurement of pulmonary wedge pressure and arterial pressure as well as very aggressive attempts to treat respiratory distress and pulmonary failure with modalities such as intubation, oxygen therapy and positive end-expiratory pressure (PEEP).

In the management of the severely bleeding patient it is essential that we consider the high degree of acuity associated with many of these patients. Such patients are generally seen in the emergency room, operating room or intensive care unit, areas somewhat unfamiliar to practitioners of blood banking. All too often, transfusion medicine specialists actually consider clinicians to be inadequate and incapable of dealing with the critical care nature of these issues. We must consider that clinicians are not necessarily idiots and that they do not always take too many risks, treat unscientifically or spend too much money in the care of their patients. Many of us in transfusion medicine have gotten used to the practice of "telephone medicine" and therefore are too far removed from the patient's bedside to recognize the critical problems that face individuals who are involved in evolving clinical situations. The incredible difficulties encountered in dealing with the bleeding patient must not be minimized when clinicians in this setting utilize such blood components as fresh frozen plasma, platelet concentrates, and cryoprecipitate to try to stop serious bleeding. It is all too easy to criticize these clinical interventions as being unscientific and too risky. However, if placed in the same situation as a clinical-care physician with an exsanguinating patient, many of us would resort to similar kinds of interventions to do whatever we think is possible to stop the bleeding.

In the arena of autologous blood donation many transfusion medicine specialists are unwilling to deal with sick patients and would prefer only dealing with the walking well. This is perhaps in keeping with our long experience with volunteer blood donors who are in fact in excellent health. But if we are to practice the profession of transfusion medicine, we must be willing to deal with sick patients even though we recognize that they may take an inordinate amount of our attention and time. They are the ones who, indeed, most likely require autologous transfusion. Many of the rules and regulations which have been promulgated in the field of autologous donation are, I believe, very much unacceptable and inappropriate. For example, we have set a minimum hematocrit for autologous blood donation, but in fact these kinds of regulations may be too restrictive and prevent our dealing with patients who need more innovative but labour intensive management. Patients with hematocrits lower than 33%, for example, may often donate 1/2 units of blood perfectly safely, which would allow for accumulations of adequate blood for upcoming surgery. Another example, is that we have set a 72 hour rule for the time of the last autologous donation until the time of surgery. This is based upon data which suggest that blood volume is not restored to normal until as long as 72 hours after a phlebotomy of 500 ml of blood. However, if we are willing to restore blood volume to normal by the infusion of volume expanders such as albumin following blood donation then, in fact, this should not be a limitation. The anesthesiologist is capable of collecting 500–1000 ml of blood or plasma immediately prior to surgery in the operating room and restoring blood volume to normal, the so called technique of acute normovolemic hemodilution. Yet blood bankers refuse to recognize that they are capable of similar kinds of manœuvers. By making didactic statements and regulations regarding the timing of preoperative collection of autologous blood, blood bankers create unacceptable limits on individualizing patient care. It is essential that transfusion medicine specialists be able to exercise good medical judgement in dealing with their patients. In this regard the use of guidelines, rather than rules and regulations would seem most appropriate and allow optimal patient care.

When dealing with the transfusion of previously collected autologous blood, again there seems to be a lack of willingness to deal with what the practice of medicine is all about. While medicine may be directed toward saving lives, much of it is also directed toward relieving pain and suffering. Therefore, when deciding whether to transfuse a patient with his own previously collected autologous blood, the use of the strict guidelines appropriate for allogenic transfusion are in no way in keeping with the recognition of the role of medicine in dealing with the postoperative patient. The relief of suffering due to weakness induced by postoperative anemia cannot be considered an inappropriate goal and is entirely analogous to the use of analgesics to reduce pain and sleeping medications to allow the patient to sleep comfortably. While the dictum of "first do no harm" must be considered, the fact is that clinical care physicians consider the relief of pain and suffering by the use of analgesics and sleeping medications to be entirely appropriate. Blood bankers have found it difficult to deal with these kinds of issues and continually recommend that patients only be transfused under life-threatening conditions. This attitude requires change.

Furthermore, blood bankers are all too often inordinately concerned with the cost-effectiveness of transfusion practices. While cost-effectiveness is of great importance, and each of us needs to be concerned with treating in a manner which is justified by the costs involved, most physicians and surgeons are willing and ready to use legitimate, newer medical strategies in dealing with the ills of their patients, irrespective of cost. We cannot continually reject newer medical therapies which in fact are safe and effective simply because we as blood bankers think they cost too much. Many patients and their clinical-care physicians do not in fact believe that the costs are inordinate given the benefits which may be derived from these therapies.

Finally, in the area of limiting donor exposure transfusion medicine physicians must make serious adjustments in their willingness to interact with donors in order to benefit critically ill patients who would profit from donor-specific components. If prospective donors are informed of the risks (which are often relatively small) engendered in frequent donation protocols, such as can be developed for limiting donor exposure, then this practice should be considered to be medically sound. While we may be correct to prohibit collection of blood from volunteer donors with hematocrits of less than 38%, we should recognize that we may benefit our patients maximally if we allow dedicated repeat donors to give at hematorcrits considerably less than this. If the patient donating autologous blood, who is often ill, can tolerate donations at levels of 33%, why then cannot his family and friends, who have a vested interest in the patient's welfare, also tolerate such kinds of donations. In this regard we must take a lesson from physicians involved in transplantation medicine. These individuals are willing to collect kidneys and bone marrow from volunteer donors who have been properly informed of the risks of these procedures in order to benefit the patient. The risks of blood donations at hematocrits of 33% or even lower are certainly less than those encountered by individuals who agree to donate a kidney or bone marrow under general anesthesia and with the dangers of a serious surgical procedure. These surgical procedures may place donors under some risk of medical complications or even death and in addition are extremely costly kinds of procedures, but are deemed to be appropriate by transplantation physicians. Transfusion medicine specialists should take a lesson from the Nobel prize-winning efforts of transplantation physicians in recognizing that proper allocation of risk and of patient-care dollars are entirely appropriate when providing significant benefits for seriously ill patients.

It seems clear to me that transfusion medicine will not be a legitimate "medical" specialty until its practitioners are willing to revert to the practices that we all learned in medical school and follow in the footsteps of our clinical colleagues by bringing our knowledge and expertise to the patient's arena of care. An unreasonable focus on cost-effectiveness can only serve to inhibit our desire to have a positive impact on patient outcome. Furthermore, didactic rules and regulations only serve to inhibit our ingenuity in dealing on an individual basis with patient-care problems. The field of transfusion medicine cannot assume clinical relevance until its practitioners are willing to mimic their clinical-care colleagues in dealing with the incredible complexity of the management of critically ill patients. Once again, the judgment of the Nobel

Prize Committee in delivering the 1990 Nobel Prize in medicine to a practitioner of bone marrow transplantation should serve as a model for transfusion medicine to focus our specialty on the needs of our patients, and be willing to assume and exercise good medical judgment in dealing with patients, donors and limited patient-care dollars. Transfusion medicine is indeed a crucial and potentially viable specialty, but it will require dedication and rededication to the needs of our patients in order to be successful.

Acknowledgements

The author thanks Samuel H. Pepkowitz, M.D. for helpful suggestions and Dianne Johnson for editorial assistance in the preparation of this manuscript. The support of the Rita and Taft Schreiber Foundation is greatly appreciated.

References

1. Goldfinger D. Acute hemolytic transfusion reactions – a fresh look at pathogenesis and considerations regarding therapy. Transfusion 1977;17:85-98.
2. Davenport RD, Strieter RM, Standiford TJ, Kunkel SL. Interleukin-8 production in red blood cell incompatibility. Blood 1990;76:2439-42.
3. Levy GJ, Shabot MM, Hart ME, Mya WW, Goldfinger D. Transfusion-associated noncardiogenic pulmonary edema. Report of a case and a warning regarding treatment. Transfusion 1986;26:278-81.

DISCUSSION

J.D. Cash, W.G. van Aken

W.G. van Aken (Amsterdam, NL): Dr. Habibi, you mentioned briefly the great disparity between the use of blood components in various countries. Do you have any suggestions how this disparity, which you think is too large, could be decreased. Could consensus conferences contribute for instance?

B. Habibi (Paris, FR): The question needs a full appraisal and long-term thought. I think the consensus meetings represent one of the ways the question may be dealt with. Indeed, both in the United States and in Europe experience shows that when clinicians, scientific professionals, blood bankers and anesthesiologists get together and look with some depth into the problem, they come out with recommendations. In hospitals we see a very important difference in the use of blood components or plasma derivatives with the same standard of patient care. That means that something must be going wrong. Experiences are numerous now to show that there is a very important effort to be concentrated on those issues. Scientific approaches, clinical studies and education of people, both blood bankers, physicians, residents, students and others must play a very important role.

J.D. Cash (Edinburgh, Scotland): I wonder at times whether, in the context of blood usage and clinical outcomes, we may have much to learn from developing countries. Later this week we will be hearing about an important initiative in this area that is going on in Europe[1]. I would like to see these studies extended over many years so that we can examine whether differences in blood usage effects patient outcomes. I have visited third world countries; the surgeons there are highly trained and one gets the impression that their perioperative morbidity and mortality in many elective surgical situations is not profoundless different from ours, yet their blood usage is very different because of its short supply.

1. Ten Duis HJ, McClelland BPL, see page 169-76.

D.B.L. McClelland (Edinburgh, Scotland): Two comments. First, these interesting audit studies such as the study that Dr. Cash was referring to, show very wide variations in practice. I think it is important to start of with a neutral hypothesis: "Let us not assume that less is always better." Dr. Goldfinger, you mentioned one possibility that a patient may actually feel better post-operatively as a result of not being grossly anemic. That is really quite important for that patient. We know virtually nothing about the relationship of post-operative hemoglobin to the outcome for the patient in the longer term after discharge, because nobody has ever asked those questions. We do have a dangerous assumption, I think, that less is always best. Second, there is now beginning to emerge from certainly two African countries that I am aware of some very important data, which may constitute the first ever genuine clinical trials of transfusion versus no transfusion. It has been possible to carry these out, because there is simply not enough blood around for all the patients. There is one study that I am aware of in grossly anemic children which has clearly demonstrated that there is a critical hemoglobin value – and it is very low – beyond which transfusion in fact does not effect mortality.

D. Goldfinger (Los Angeles, CA, USA): If I can make a comment on the issue of the use of too many blood components. In our own hospital we have seen the same kind of problems I am sure many of you have. In the use of platelet transfusions we are seeing an unbelievable number of platelets being given today. Very often in a patient with leukemia we see a daily or even sometimes more frequently than daily transfusion of platelets. We all tend to think when we come to meetings like this that perhaps that is an inappropriate use of platelet transfusion. I am sure many of these patients would survive without it. I remember when platelet transfusions were really not available or only very minimally available, that a lot of leukemic patients used to bleed to death. Perhaps we are really doing something good. It is impossible for us to know ahead of time exactly which patients might do well without those transfusions. Perhaps clinicians are not so wrong in administering these transfusions, because they are seeing the same kind of things. We remember that patients used to bleed to death, now they are no longer doing so. One approach that we have chosen to take is that if we cannot stop them from transfusing, how about giving safer products. For example the use of single donor platelet apheresis concentrates rather than multiple units of platelets harvested from units of whole blood. I think that giving safer components rather than simply trying to reduce the number of transfusions that we administer might be a watchword for the next ten years.

C.F. Högman (Uppsala, SW): When I listen to this discussion, I recall that many years ago Dr. J.P. Allain[1] showed an exponential dose-response curve

---

1. Allain JP. Dose requirement for replacement therapy in hemophilia. A Thromb Haemost 1979;42:825-31.

concerning the treatment of hemophilia with increasing doses of factor VIII. The use of one IU factor VIII per inhabitant has an enormous impact because you avoid the most serious effects of the factor VIII deficiency. The more you use, the more the curve bends, indicating a poorer dose-response. When you increase the dose from 3 to 4 IU per inhabitant, the therapeutical improvement is thus less impressive but the cost and need of factor VIII is strongly increased. The problem is who shall decide what is enough. Apparently, there is a different view, because some countries claim that they manage quite well with two units per inhabitant for their hemophiliacs. But when we discuss these things with our clinicians using 4.5 IU per inhabitant, they simply deny that they would overuse factor VIII. They say: We feel that we treat our patients in a very good way. So, how would a blood banker tell his colleague that he is wrong. I do not think I could. We could try to reach at a consensus about optimum. Another example concerns platelet concentrates, as you just brought up. My feeling is that when we switched from traditional platelet concentrates to leukocyte-depleted platelet concentrates, we really achieved something. Nowadays our patients are more seldom refractory to treatment, because we simply do not immunize them and they do not form HLA-antibodies any longer. So, this I think is another example of what we can achieve by improving the quality of our products. It is our concern, because we take up new technology and we can communicate with our clinical colleagues. The consensus would be that we have a good communication with our clinical colleagues.

B. Habibi: Thank you Dr. Högman for your remarks. I think that humility is the first point we should keep in mind in that kind of discussion. However, I think the only way to handle those uncertainties is to get scientific data, to have clinical investigations done and to found our recommendations on scientific grounds. That is important, otherwise you cannot solve any problem.

C.Th. Smit Sibinga (Groningen, NL): Dr. Wagstaff, within the policy setting and making authorities there is a shift noticeable to a specific aspect of the transfusion practice regarding the products blood banks produce out of the human blood as a tissue: Being medicinal products. I can see that being legitimate for as long as it relates to the processing per se, the GMP aspects. But having it carried over the boundaries of GMP into the clinic and actually destining blood components and derivatives to just a medicine or an infusate, I think goes beyond the factual practice of blood transfusion at the bedside. For as far as the concept relates to the safety, the purity and the potency of blood components and derivatives it is all ok, but there is also the clinical efficacy. Could you give your comments?

W. Wagstaff (Sheffield, UK): Sure, I agree with you entirely. The concept that blood and its products and components were to be regarded in the same light as pharmaceutical products was something that was completely alien to us when first introduced in the EC Directive in 1985. I think that many of us still find it difficult to accept this. particularly, from the point you made in the latter part of the question. Although we can follow the lines of trying to produce safe products, it is almost impossible to dictate in advance just how effective these products are going to be, because of the intrinsic biological variation. My personal point of view is that if the lawyers in Brussels dictate that this is what we must do, then so be it. It just so happens that we benefit from this dictation in as much as it is focused on a subject which we have neglected for too long. Most of us have nodded in the direction of quality control of the old style for a long time, but really have not structured thoughts until this new legislation was imposed on us. I agree entirely with you; it maybe totally inappropriate to regard products in this fashion, but on the other hand I think it does really help us to go from here onwards, to produce safer if not completely effective products.

F. Peetoom (Portland, OR, USA): As many of you probably have heard the American Red Cross is reorganizing its manufacturing process. The focus is to basically follow all the principles that we heard presented by Dr. Wagstaff. I had the feeling that he followed a training course at the FDA, because we are indeed using all those same terms and use the same language to instill into our staffs the following of this new manufacturing process, its documentation and so forth. Then, there are the doctor Goldfingers in the Red Cross also, who feel indeed that this becomes a tremendous imposition on the ability to provide service, that needs to be customized in many instances. The absoluteness of many of those rules and the severity of punishment by breaking those rules, make it seem difficult to do something that we feel belongs to the practice of medicine and clinical service. So, the next development in response to this concern is that the American national Red Cross is looking at an organizational division between the manufacturing process per se and all those products and services that do have to be segregated from the single standard and uniformity of the manufacturing of procedures. These would then be able to continue in a clinical service's setting and would be a different part of the organization which is represented at a national, separate level and also at the regional levels. In fact we would then be able to preserve some of those special services like the mother with a hematocrit of 37 who might want to give blood for her child, which currently is not allowed in the FDA regulations. I am not sure how we work this out with the Food and Drug Administration, but we are trying to maintain the opportunity for innovation and individualized services that make practical medical sense without running into trouble with the FDA regulations.

W. Wagstaff: Dr. Peetoom, I think I understood the imminent division that you are talking about. I am not sure that I whole heartedly agree with that, to be honest, because I think that if there is an attempt made to complete this, segregating the manufacturing side of our business (and I use the word advisedly) from the clinical side, then what may tend to happen is that all of the components produced by a conventional transfusion centre now may be governed by the same sort of pharmacological strict rules that govern fractionated plasma components. Eventually you may see the situation whereby, not just for the manufacturing processes but for the end-products as well, the standards may be set by people who are by training more accustomed to producing aspirin than to treating patients. My own view is that the logical thing would be to maintain the medical input as well as the scientific in the setting of your manufacturing standards, so that you can reach some sort of balance between what is achievable and what is best for the patient. But at the same time achievable from the donor population which in itself is subject to such variation. The pure manufacturing process tends to lose sight of the vageries of the raw materials that we are dealing with and may set standards which are so high in fact as to be restrictive with regard to what can be done by the clinicians at the other end.

A. Heaton (Norfolk, VA, USA): I think that the move toward good manufacturing practices will affect not only the issue of transfusion medicine, but also the future of physicians within blood banking. In the American Red Cross the upcoming new president is going to be from the pharmaceutical industry, not an MD. That reflects the American Red Cross's perspectives on the way the future is going. In fact: I think we are going to have a split between blood production and transfusion medicine that may affect the survival of physicians as managers in the blood bank. If you are a physician in the blood bank you may be involved in the transfusion medicine end of the profession, whereas if you are not a physician you may well be involved only in the production process. This would be possible if each donor was treated as a biological manufacturing plant and therefore the requirement was GMP type standards to the donation process. So, in the future, it may not be economically viable to have a physician in charge of a blood bank, as it would be illogical to spend that much money on a very expensive person who requires a long-training, when in fact you could hire a very much less expensive administrative type of pharmacist to drive your production plant and then to use your physician exclusively in the area of transfusion medicine à la the Goldfinger approach. Under this approach the physician's expertise would be used to customize the product and meet patients' needs. So, for me this whole issue of transfusion medicine is really going to be the future of doctors in blood banking, because as I see it, blood banking is going to be rapidly split into the production of standardized products as one subspecialty and transfusion medicine as a second specialty which will diverge from the former over the years.

B.T. Teague (Houston, TX, USA): I believe there is a lot of merit to what you say, but I think that there are two areas of concern. If I had a red flag to run up to say: "Danger, think more about this", I would run it up right now. Being aware of generalizing both in statistics and the way people are treated, we have a tendency to look at statistics and say that per capita there is so many of this, either in transfusion or donations. But in fact if you tear those apart and look at single patients within that usage, there are very bonafide reasons why one patient may need more than another. There are very bonafide reasons why some donations may be less and yet just as effective under certain circumstances. So, I would caution against the generalization with statistics. The other item that I think relates to this, is cost effectiveness or cost economics. As Dr. Goldfinger has indicated, no one has really defined that. Frankly I believe that it is probably more economical to convert to platelets from apheresis to reduce infectious disease transmission than it is to either treat a case of transfusion transmitted AIDS or significant hepatitis and include the loss of productivity in that particular individual. It may be even more economical to convert to platelets from apheresis than it is to spend money on one loss that would resolve from someone thinking that wrong had been done. So, I get concerned when there are generalizations made and not specifics and I go back to the customer service aspect. If in fact the physician believes that that decision on their part is the best for that patient, I believe that you need to fill that particular order, whatever it may be. In the event that it does cost more, I think that will work itself out, but you can justify quality service in patient care as the bottom line.

II. REGULATORY AND LEGAL ASPECTS

TRANSFUSION MEDICINE: THE ROLE OF THE LAW

J.K.M. Gevers

Introduction

The role of the law in health care is an important one. A modern health care system cannot exist without a considerable amount of legal regulation. There is so much at stake for society and its members if that system does not function properly, that there is no society that does not want to exert power over its health care system. In a democratic society the law is an appropriate instrument to establish such control. Has the law a particular role to play with regard to transfusion medicine? If we look at the legislation of many nations in the world, the answer would seem to be affirmative. There is no issue of the International Digest of Health Legislation for instance – a periodical of the WHO which provides a comprehensive survey of national health legislation – in which you would not find abstracts of new laws or regulations in the field of blood transfusion. Apparently, transfusion medicine is considered an area which deserves legal regulation. This is not surprising: the fact that blood and blood products are administered to patients as therapeutic substances in itself already justifies at least some legal control. The human origin of these substances and their natural scarcity are further reasons for interference by society and the legislator.

The question to discuss is, which objectives the law on transfusion medicine should serve and how it could be shaped to reach those objectives. In answering these questions, I will first focus on the underlying principles; subsequently, I will try to set out some basic elements of transfusion law and discuss briefly different ways in which these elements could be incorporated in the law. Finally, I will say a few words on the issue of harmonization since one cannot discuss national transfusion law without at least touching upon the international aspects. As to the facts and fictions: I will address that theme briefly in my conclusions.

Legal principles

First of all the principles which are at the basic of the law concerning blood transfusion. Three groups of principles can be distinguished [1].

The first group comprises the right to self-determination and the rights to protection of physical integrity and privacy. These are fundamental human rights, embodied in international treaties and national constitutions. They were not specifically developed with a view to the health care sector of course, but over the last decades their relevance to the practice of medicine has been recognized to an ever growing extent. Their implications for transfusion medicine are obvious. Self-determination means voluntariness with regard to both the donation and the reception of blood. No pressure must be brought to bear upon a donor; it should be his own decision whether or not to serve the interests of others by donating blood. The patient needing blood is free to refuse it, even if in doing so he would act against his own interest as perceived by his doctor or by others. The protection of physical integrity and privacy requires informed consent for the medical acts needed to collect blood and to administer it, and confidentiality of the personal medical data generated in the process.

The second group of principles is associated with the so called social right to health care. That right entails a responsibility of the public authorities to protect and promote the health of the population and therefore to take the necessary steps in safeguarding the availability, accessibility, quality and safety of health care services. It goes without saying that principles such as equal access and protection of quality and safety are of paramount importance in a domain such as transfusion medicine, taking into account the natural scarcity of blood and the dangers inherent in its use.

Finally a third category of basic norms should be mentioned, related to blood as a substance of human origin: the principles of non-remuneration, self-sufficiency and optimal use of the limited supply for medical or related purposes. Although these principles are less general than the fundamental rights mentioned before, they are not specific for the blood transfusion. The ongoing developments in the field of transplantation have increased their importance also for the collection and use of other kinds of human cells and tissues, and therefore for transplantation medicine as a whole. Principles like non-remuneration and self-sufficiency are not legal principles in a strict sense; usually, ethical, clinical and public policy reasons are given to support them. In my opinion, also these principles should be incorporated firmly in the law, including international legal instruments, as they are of crucial importance, now and in the future, for transplantation medicine in general.

Elements of transfusion law

Against this background, what should be the basic elements of national transfusion law? Let us first look at the objectives. In my opinion the law in this domain should have at least four aims:

- to lay down the principle of non-remuneration in blood donation and to prevent commercial exploitation;
- to provide a legal framework to promote self-sufficiency and to ensure optimal use of blood for medical purposes;
- to protect the donor in terms of autonomy, physical integrity and privacy;
- to protect recipients in terms of quality, safety and accessibility of services.

Taking into account these aims, many aspects can be mentioned which should be covered – in one way or another – by national transfusion law. International declarations, such as the Code of Ethics of the International Society of Blood Transfusion (adopted in 1980 in Montreal and approved by the League of Red Cross Societies) [2,3] and the Recommendation on the responsibilities of health authorities in the field of blood transfusion (adopted by the Council of Europe in 1988) [4] provide ample guidance on this point.

As to the first objective, the law should ensure that donors do not obtain financial benefit from giving blood and that the collection of blood and plasma is entrusted only to non-profit-making agencies; at the same time, the donor must be left in no doubt that donations are being used for patients in need without financial gain for any intermediate party.

The second objective (self-sufficiency and optimal use) requires a legal framework providing for the existence of a coordinated network of blood transfusion services. According to the Council of Europe Recommendation of 1988, a national program should be established covering the different stages of transfusion and meeting medical needs concerning blood and blood products [4]. The law should say who bears the responsibility for collection, preparation, preservation and distribution of blood. It should designate the agencies which may act as transfusion services, protect their activities (for instance through a system of licensing) and make provision for the assessment of proficiency and quality of these services. Furthermore, the law should set out the conditions under which importation or exportation of blood or blood products would be allowed.

As to the third objective (protection of the donor), first of all the law should ensure that no coercion or pressure be brought to bear on a potential donor and that donors be advised of the risks connected with the collection of blood. Blood should be collected under the responsibility of a physician. When procedures are carried out which entail increased risks for a donor (such as plasma- or cytapheresis), he must be informed of the additional risks and adequate measures must be taken for his protection. Donors must be adequately informed about the measures adopted with regard to donor selection, such as the screening of donated blood on infectious agents. Legal safeguards should exist concerning the confidentiality of all personal donor details, including the results of all laboratory tests. I would like to emphasize, that confidentiality surrounding blood donations is not only required by every citizen's right to privacy, but is also a cornerstone of a system of voluntary blood donation.

Finally, the law should ensure that adequate compensation will be paid in the event of complications related to the taking of blood, for instance by requiring that such events should be covered by insurance.

As to the fourth objective (the protection of recipients) the international declarations mentioned before require several measures to be taken to reach this objective. The law should first of all ensure that suitable testing of each donor and blood donation be performed in order to detect abnormalities that are likely to be harmful to recipients; for this purpose transfusion services should have detailed criteria for donor selection and deferral. Secondly, the law should make provision for internal and external quality control throughout all the stages of the transfusion process. These provisions should relate to the proficiency of staff, the adequacy of the equipment and premises, and the quality of methods, reagents and final products. When blood or blood products are imported from other countries, the law should make provisions for arrangements ensuring the quality and safety of these substances or of the source materials used in their preparation. Finally, concerning the actual transfusion, the law should ensure that all patients can benefit from the administration of human blood or blood products whatever their financial resources, and that it takes place carefully under the responsibility of a physician so as to protect the safety of the patient.

The nature of transfusion law

Until now, the main principles, objectives and elements of transfusion law have been briefly delineated. A further question is, how these elements should be incorporated in national law. Should there be a single act covering all these aspects or should an eventual transfusion act be limited to what is specific in the collection, preparation and administration of blood and blood products and refer to more general health care legislation for other aspects? Should a blood transfusion act contain detailed regulations and give most power and responsibilities to the central authorities, or should it rather be more indirect in character, leaving regulation of the details to the agencies operating in this field?

So far as the first question is concerned, we should realize that in most countries many elements of transfusion medicine are already covered by more general health law. this holds in particular for the protection of the donor and the recipient. Normally, medical acts like the taking of blood and its administration will come under the laws covering the medical profession and under malpractice and disciplinary law. The rights of the donor to adequate information on blood collection procedures, the informed consent and the confidentiality of personal data, will usually be protected, at least in a general way, by laws on patient rights or on privacy protection. The laws on medical drugs and devices, and even general laws on the licensing of health care facilities may include provisions on quality assurance which are of relevance to the safety of the recipients of blood and blood products.

It is obvious, that in designing national transfusion law one must take account of the potential overlap with other health care legislation and refrain from regulating elements which have already been adequately covered by other laws. In my opinion, a separate act on blood transfusion will usually be appropriate but it should focus on the elements which are typical for transfusion medicine (such as prevention of commercialization, the establishment of a national program and of a network of qualified agencies designated to carry it out; regulation of import and export, etc.), with additional provisions on other elements such as the position of the donor, but only to the extent that general laws do not give sufficient protection.

Why not embody the law on blood transfusion in a general transplantation law, encompassing also other transplants such as bone marrow, tissue and organs? This would have the advantage that a number of elements which need to be regulated in all forms of transplantation (the principle of non-commercialization and self-sufficiency; the licensing and control of agencies engaged in the collection, preparation and distribution of substances of human origin; additional provisions to protect potential donors), can be laid down in one single act. It should be noted, however, that this possibility has also its drawbacks taking into account the considerable differences between the practice of transfusion medicine and other forms of transplantation, in particular if vital organs like hearts, lungs and kidneys are concerned.

An important question in legislating transfusion medicine is whether a transfusion act should be direct or indirect in its approach and to what extent it should be exhaustive in regulating transfusion practice. It is hard to give a general answer to that question, since much will depend on the characteristics and traditions of both the national legal system and the health care system. In some countries the central authorities may be given direct and extensive responsibilities including powers to enact more detailed regulations, while in others, the law may limit itself to laying down basic principles, organizational arrangements and safeguards to ensure that medical practice meets accepted standards and that the guidelines issued in accordance with the law are effectively respected. There is a tendency in health legislation to adopt the second alternative and to prefer framework laws rather than very detailed and comprehensive legislation. The developments in the fields of science and technology are going too fast and modern health care systems are becoming too complex for the legislator to elaborate regulations on all technical and organizational aspects and to keep those regulations up to date.

As far as legislation in the Netherlands is concerned, it is remarkable that our new Blood Transfusion Act, which was adopted in 1988 and which since then has only partially come into force, is still based on a rather centralistic model in which the public authorities are given substantive tasks and responsibilities. The Act has been criticized for this approach. Rightly so, in my view, although it makes provision for a national advisory body with wide terms of reference and with a broad composition including representatives of transfusion services and laboratories, donors and patients, the medical profession, hospitals and insurers.

Harmonization of transfusion law?

As said before, it is impossible to discuss national transfusion law without saying at least a few words about the international aspects. At first sight this may not be obvious, taking into account the prominent place of the principle of national self-sufficiency. However, since the achievement of a lasting balance between supply and need can never be relied on, national law should leave at least some room for import and export. Furthermore, with respect to one or more blood products, countries may want to cooperate and to increase international exchanges. Countries may even try to achieve self-sufficiency on the regional, rather than on the national level. The Council of Europe recommendation on plasma products, adopted in 1990, for instance, exhorts national health authorities "to cooperate closely to achieve European self-sufficiency in the framework of the European Economic Community and the Council of Europe" [5]; the European Economic Community directive of 1989 on medicinal products derived from human blood or human plasma talks in Article 3, section 4 about "Community self-sufficiency in human blood or human plasma" and states that, in order to achieve that purpose, member states shall encourage the voluntary unpaid donation of blood and plasma [6].

One aspect of international cooperation is its consequences for national transfusion law and in particular the need for harmonization. Different levels of harmonization may be distinguished. At the most basic level, in order to facilitate international exchange of blood and blood products the existence of common technical standards is required, for instance concerning Good Manufacturing Practice or the selection of donors. When further cooperation is envisaged, in particular if self-sufficiency at regional level is aimed at, consensus is needed on underlying basic principles such as non-remuneration of blood donors. If one wants to establish a common market all obstacles to trade have to be removed so that manufacturers can be assured that when their product meets commonly defined standards, it will be accepted on the internal market of all member states without discrimination. It is exactly the objective of the already mentioned EEC directive of 1989 to achieve such a degree of harmonization with regard to industrially prepared blood products, in particular albumin, coagulation factors and immunoglobulins of human origin.

It goes without saying that the ongoing efforts towards harmonization, in particular when harmonization measures are legally binding upon countries as the EEC directives are, have immediate consequences for national law. It is not unlikely, for instance, that the new Dutch Blood Transfusion Act of 1988, which contains rather strict requirements with respect to imports of blood products, will have to be amended in order to bring it in accordance with the EEC directive on that subject. In fact, the EEC directive was elaborated after the proposal for the Blood Transfusion Bill was notified by the Dutch authorities to the European Economic Community; that notification took place in pursuance of an obligatory information procedure adopted by the community in 1983, which since 1987 applies also to national draft legislation regarding blood products. Harmonization directives in the European Economic Community are adopted by a majority vote. Although a high level of protection is aimed at by the European Commission, member states have to remain on the alert as to whether such directives meet the level of safety and health protection they want to achieve for their citizens; once a directive has been adopted, there is hardly any room left for exceptions at national level. Some observers have expressed concern, that the directive on blood products with its primarily economic objective of removal of trade barriers may open the door to commercialization and may therefore in the long run result in less than optimal protection for blood recipients.

Conclusions

In concluding, let me say by way of summary that to some extent, legal regulation of transfusion medicine is indispensable. It is the responsibility of national authorities to elaborate appropriate legislation and to enforce it where necessary. In shaping legal arrangements at national level, several factors have to be taken into account, such as the extent to which the field is already covered by other laws and the nature of the existing national legal and health care system. Therefore, it is impossible to delineate one single, common model for national laws on blood transfusion. On the other hand the international exchange of blood products calls for a minimum of harmonization.

What about the facts and fictions?

While recognizing the importance of legislation, we should remain aware of its inherent limitations. Sometimes politicians, lawyers, but also health professionals seem to believe, that good law is a guarantee for good practice and that the law is a perfect instrument to control social processes or to bring about social change. In legislating transfusion medicine, one should avoid this pitfall. The legislator cannot comprehensively regulate the complex reality of modern blood transfusion. The field of transfusion medicine is a dynamic one; the law cannot control it completely, let alone anticipate future developments. Very often, laws fall short of their ends or have undesirable side effects; laws are never completely up to date. The fact that they are not always complied with and remain unenforced, can sometimes even be a blessing in disguise. That is exactly why the method of "indirect" legislation is often preferred nowadays. While remaining loyal to its underlying principles and its objectives, the law should serve the practice of transfusion medicine and support progress rather than frustrating it. This means that good transfusion law will not be made by politicians and lawyers alone, but in a continuous dialogue with those working in the field of blood transfusion.

38

References

1. Jonker H, de Bijl N. Enkele juridische aspecten van het bloedtransfusievraagstuk. T Soc Gezondheidszorg 1988;66:96-100.
2. International Society of Blood Transfusion. Code of ethics for blood donation and transfusion. Int Dig of Health Legislation 1981;32:170-3.
3. League of Red Cross and Red Crescent Societies. Statement on the ethics of voluntary, non-remunerated blood donation. Int Dig of Health Legislation 1991;42: 175-6.
4. Council of Europe. Recommendation No. R(88)4 on the responsibilities of health authorities in the field of blood transfusion. Int Dig of Health Legistlation 1989;40: 69-72.
5. Council of Europe. Recommendation No. R(90)9 on plasma products and European self-sufficiency. Int Dig of Health Legislation 1991;42:27-30.
6. European Communities. Council directive of 14 June 1989 on medicinal products derived from human blood or human plasma. Off J Eur Communities 1989;L181: 44-6.

REGULATIONS AND REGULATORY MECHANISMS RELATED TO TRANSFUSION MEDICINE IN THE UNITED STATES OF AMERICA

J.S. Epstein

Introduction

History of US regulation of drugs and biologics

In the United States of America (US), federal regulation of blood-related products began with "therapeutic serum" defined under the Virus, Serum and Toxins Act of 1902, which was passed in response to an occurrence of tetanus contaminated diphtheria anti-toxin. Subsequently, in reaction to shocking public disclosures of worthless and dangerous patient medications, the US Congress passed the Food and Drug Act of 1906. This law provided the first legal definition of a drug subject to regulation, and declared that drugs distributed in interstate commerce may not be misbranded, adulterated, poisonous or deleterious. Additional authority to regulate blood and blood products was derived by consideration of blood as a drug under this act, although this indirect authority was later successfully contested in court.

Following 107 deaths due to contamination of Elixir of sulfanilamide, the Federal Food, Drug and Cosmetic Act (FD&C Act) of 1938 was enacted, establishing the need for manufacturers to demonstrate drug safety before marketing, and providing a broader definition of a drug. This act was amended in 1962, following the thalidomide tragedy in Europe, to increase the assurance of safety prior to commercialization and to require that drug manufacturers demonstrate drug effectiveness as well as safety. Provisions of the FD&C Act included definition of Good Manufacturing Practices, requirements for annual registration of manufacturers and biennial inspections. In 1976, the Medical Device Amendments to the FD&C Act extended regulatory authority for assurance of safety and efficacy to include medical devices.

In 1944, the Public Health Services (PHS) Act unified and codified the regulation of biologic products. Blood products were not specifically identified as biologic products under the PHS Act until passage of an amendment in 1973. Also in 1972, the jurisdiction for regulation of blood products was transferred from the National Institutes of Health to the Food and Drug Administration (FDA). Soon thereafter, in 1976, the FDA published specific regulations governing blood and source plasma collection establishments. The evolution of the US federal government involvement in regulation of medical products, including blood and blood products, shaped the principles that still govern its regulatory philosophy. The need for regulation was established by the abuses of the past which occurred for lack of restraints on manufacturers operating in free market. As a result, the concept of premarket validation has been established, including the demonstration of both safety and efficacy. Blood and blood components for transfusion and source plasma intended for manufacturing into injectable plasma derivatives are identified as biologic products under the PHS Act. The regulations which have been put in place related to these products serve to protect the public health and safety by defining acceptable manufacturing practices at all levels from donor selection and screening, through product manufacturing and labelling, to record keeping. The mechanisms by which this is accomplished are described in this manuscript.

Structure of the blood system in the US

As a background for a discussion of regulatory mechanisms, it may be useful to describe the blood system in the US. First, it must be recognized that blood products and services are provided by the private sector, either as commercial or non-profit enterprises, in contrast to the national transfusion services which operate in many other counties. The fact of privatization leads to the need for strong and effective regulation to maintain a uniform national standard of quality, despite a large and diverse political and economic system.

A second basic fact is the distinction between collection of whole blood and components for transfusion vs. source plasma for fractionation. Blood and components for transfusion are obtained from unpaid volunteers, whereas source plasma is obtained by apheresis primarily from paid donors. Collections of whole blood from paid donors also occur for the purpose of making *in vitro* diagnostic reagents. Since 1978, blood must be labelled to reflect either a volunteer or paid donor. Plasma recovered from volunteer whole blood collection also may be released for fractionation as "recovered plasma", however, this constitutes only approximately 20% of the source material which is processed into plasma derivatives.

Annually, whole blood is obtained from approximately eight million donors who provide 12.5 million collections (i.e. an average of 1.5 donations per year). In any year, about 20% of blood collections are from first time donors, and 60% are from males. Autologous donations represent 2-10% of the current blood supply. A more accurate current estimate for the contribution of autologous collections is lacking because of the recent increases in self-donation in the AIDS era, especially since 1988. The FDA registers and inspects approximately 2,300 blood establishments. This number includes approximately 200 establishments operating at roughly 400 locations which produce products intended for distribution in interstate commerce, and which have licensing requirements. Within this system, the American Red Cross (ARC) operates in 50 regions at more than 250 facilities under a single license. Collections by the ARC represent approximately 50% of the US supply of whole blood and components for transfusion. Most laboratory testing of whole blood and components is performed on-site at fixed establishments, while as much as two thirds or more of collections may occur on mobile units.

Annually, approximately one million donors provide ten million collections of source plasma which result in seven million litres for fractionation. An additional two million litres of "recovered plasma" are released for fractionation, 60% by the ARC. Approximately three million litres of US source plasma are used in Europe. Over 99% of the donors of source plasma receive payment. There are approximately 70 licensed establishments which operate at about 450 locations. These facilities employ 10,000 people in 200 cities located in 42 states. Eighty percent of them are owned by five companies. Approximately 90% of the screening tests are performed off-site by ten reference laboratories.

A total of 20 manufacturers are licensed to make and distribute plasma derivatives. Approximately 30 additional manufacturers are approved to make diagnostic test kits for infectious disease screening and blood grouping reagents. More than 90 establishments are registered to make medical devices related to blood collection and processing. This includes collection containers and component separation devices which are regulated as medical devices.

A third basic concept is that FDA regulation is focused on the activities of the product manufacturer and not on the use of products by physicians. Manufacturers are held accountable for maintaining proper facilities, for carrying

Table 1. Regulatory mechanisms related to FDA authority over blood and blood products.

Area of FDA authority	Regulation mechanism
Approvals	Establishment licensing
	Product licensing and approval
Surveillance	Establishment registration
	Establishment inspections
	Error and accident reports
	Product testing
	Phase IV studies
	Lot release
Enforcement	Regulatory actions
Communication of policy	Regulations
	Guidelines
	Points to consider
	Memoranda to establishments
	Letters to establishments
	Advisory committee

out appropriate manufacturing procedures and for providing complete and truthful labels. The FDA does not regulate the medical use of the products except by determining what is allowed in a manufacturer's product claim.

Regulatory mechanisms related to transfusion medicine

The basic FDA regulatory mechanisms related to blood products are summarized in Table 1. The Agency's activities related to these mechanisms are summarized in Table 2.

Approval authorities related to establishments and products

FDA regulation of the nation's blood system operates through approval authorities related both to the establishments and the products. All blood collection establishments must register annually with the FDA. In addition, it is necessary to obtain a license prior to manufacturing products which are intended for distribution in interstate commerce. Both registered facilities and licensed establishments must comply with all the applicable regulations issued by the FDA.

The objective of FDA review of establishment applications prior to issuance of a license is to insure that current Good Manufacturing Practices (GMPs) are in place. Elements of the establishment review for GMPs include assessment of the physical structure, management responsibility, personnel training, plant safety and security, handling systems for water and air, environmental monitoring for organisms and particulates, and waste management including

Table 2. FDA activities related to regulation of blood establishments and products.

Mechanism of regulation	Related activities
Establishment licensing	Facility review (GMPs) Pre-license inspection
Product approval	Manufacturing review Review of preclinical and clinical data Labelling review
Surveillance	Review of reports and inspectional findings Determination of violations Health hazard evaluation Case management

Enforcement	Regulatory actions
	     Warning letters
	     Seizures and recalls
	     License suspensions and revocations
	 Court mediated actions
	     Injunctions
	     Prosecution

special handling of toxic wastes. A review of Standard Operating Procedures (SOPs) is carried out to determine whether they comply with all existing regulations and recommendations.

For each licensed establishment, the FDA also reviews product applications for each of the blood products which will be manufactured. This review primarily confirms that procedures and product labelling are in accordance with published regulations and guidelines for recognized products. Only new products or indications require extensive submission of data for review. Guidelines and recommendations already exist regarding most aspects of product manufacturing for whole blood, blood components and source plasma. Specifically, the FDA has regulated donor selection criteria, donor testing, phlebotomy procedures, product manufacturing, product labelling and record keeping related both to donor and product histories.

For manufacturers of other injectable blood products, such as plasma derivatives, as well as for manufacturers of test kits and reagents used to insure the safety of blood products, the FDA review also includes a detailed assessment of manufacturing procedures to insure identity, purity, potency and stability of all components, and to validate the adequacy of quality control tests. In recent years, validation of viral inactivation during manufacturing of clotting factor concentrates has been closely examined. Extensive use is made of clinical trials prior to commercial approval in order to demonstrate product safety and efficacy and to validate product claims. The pre-license review also includes product labelling and advertising.

Surveillance and enforcement authorities

In addition to establishment and product approvals, the FDA maintains both active and passive surveillance to insure compliance with regulatory requirements and standards. Active surveillance includes on-site inspections which, since 1988, are performed annually rather than biennially for all registered establishments. Also, licensees are required to report all errors and accidents, and all establishments must report transfusion associated deaths. For plasma derivatives and diagnostic reagents, the FDA also maintains a program of lot-by-lot product testing or intermittent surveillance testing using reference reagents or procedures which are standardized by FDA scientists. Product lots which fail FDA testing may not be commercially distributed.

In response to reports of errors and accidents, or inspectional findings, the FDA carries out an assessment to identify violations of its standards and any associated health hazard. Unsuitable products which were released in violation of FDA standards are subject to recalls which are monitored by the Agency. In urgent situations, the FDA may seize and take control of the products. Based on the potential public health impact of documented violations, additional legal actions may be taken by the Agency. These include issuance of warning letters, license suspensions and revocations, obtaining of court injunctions and criminal prosecution.

Communication and development of regulatory policies

Communication with the blood industry occurs through publication of regulations, guidelines, points to consider, memoranda and letters to establishments. Regulations, which have the force of law, are published in Title 21 of the US Code of Federal Regulations. Generally, it takes years to develop and publish regulations due to an elaborate process of revisions including the opportunity for public comment.

Guidelines, which are announced in the Federal Register, are position statements by the Agency which clarify its interpretations and expectations related to published regulations. Adherence to guidelines provides blood establishments with legal protection since the guidelines define the activities that FDA regards as compliant with regulation. Points to consider, also announced in the Federal Register, identify the issues which the Agency will examine in relation to establishment or product license application reviews.

Compared with regulations, the publication of memoranda and letters to establishments are more rapid and flexible methods by which the FDA can define industry standards. Recommendations made by memoranda and letters can be enforced when they become part of an establishment's SOPs.

The authority for promulgation of regulations related to blood and blood products rests with the FDA commissioner. In the present FDA structure, blood product issues are managed either in the Division of Transfusion Science or the Division of Hematology of the FDA's Center for Biologic Evaluation and Research. The Center Director may issue recommendations in the form of guidelines, points to consider and memoranda. Significant developments in policy are usually discussed at meetings of a scientific advisory committee. These meetings are open to the public, although closed sessions may be utilized for discussion of proprietary issues with the FDA advisors. The Agency also participates as a liaison member to various groups in the private sector which are engaged in the development of voluntary standards.

The concept of a review scientist is basic to policy development at the FDA. In all of its administrative activities, an effort is made to insure that policy development is responsive to current science, as interpreted by resident experts and outside consultants. The need to maintain research expertise was recognized historically in the area of biologic products and remains appropriate in the face of the sweeping innovations due to biotechnology. For blood products, technology change has included the development of recombinant-DNA derived products such as growth factors like erythropoietin, eventual substitutes for naturally derived injectable products, such as Factor VIII, new pharmacologic agents related to natural substances, such as tPA, and the use of neoantigens and monoclonal antibodies as diagnostic reagents. Issues related to determination of product safety and efficacy have often required laboratory experimentation. Control of infectious risks related to HIV has also required epidemiologic surveillance, for example to define risk factors used as a basis for donor deferral, and behavioral research to improve the communication between blood establishments and prospective donors.

New trends in FDA regulation of blood establishments

1. Quality assurance management

In the last decade, the development of standards appropriate to control of hepatitis and HIV transmission has resulted in dramatic changes in the blood system, including the expanded use of medical and behavioral risk histories, increased sophistication in the use of voluntary donor deferral, and an increase in the number of tests performed on collections. Furthermore, there are broadened responsibilities of blood establishments for education and counselling of donors both before and after testing.

In this context, an increased emphasis is now being placed on overall quality assurance management. This focus is a natural and progressive outgrowth of the increased complexity of blood center operations. As with other therapeutic agents, the safety of blood products depends on the accuracy, consistency and accountability of all parts of the system that produces them. It has been observed that manufacturing errors and violations of FDA standards often result from an incomplete quality management approach which results in lack of operational control.

To reduce errors and accidents, the FDA seeks to define the elements of an adequate quality assurance program and then to provide a guidance document to blood establishments. Issues to be defined include the principles of management for quality, the methods for foolproofing and error handling, techniques of monitoring (including inspections, record audits, random sampling and proficiency testing), identification of key areas for quality assurance management (including donor selection, computer software validation, labelling and tracking, testing, worker training and materials processing) and proper application of GMPs to the specific procedures of blood collection and processing.

Advances in equipment automation and computerized data management may result in improved product safety through reduced impact of human error. However, care is needed in validating such systems to prevent them from causing automatic and repetitive errors. In the area of computer software, the FDA has recognized a need to develop guidance which would define the parameters of an adequate system and a standard method of validation.

The FDA also seeks to facilitate compliance with regulations by making more readily available the check lists and criteria which inspectors should apply. Also, the Agency is seeking to expedite the publication of regulations and recommendations which will assist blood establishments in implementing standard control measures.

2. Donor related issues

Improving the efficacy of donor deferral to prevent collection of units from donors at risk for transmission of infectious diseases is a second area of intense activity. Voluntary deferral has been valuable in reducing the transfusion risks of HIV, hepatitis and malaria. Further improvement is sought in the use of donor education, communication and deferral to reduce the remaining risk of HIV transmission. Approximately 80% of male donors and approximately 60% of female donors found to be seropositive for HIV have risk factors that should have led to voluntary deferral [1]. An opportunity therefore exists to modify the interaction between blood establishments and donors so as to reduce or eliminate continued donations by persons at recognizable risk. The FDA has invested heavily in behavioral research to develop improved communication strategies for the blood establishment-donor interaction.

Related to this initiative is an effort to optimize the use of deferral registries. The Agency is placing increasing emphasis on the need for computerized data bases which will reliably identify collections from previously deferred persons, whether based on risk histories or the results of previous testing. Attempts are also being made to encourage more frequent donations by persons at lower risk for sexually transmitted diseases.

3. New product approvals

Approval of safe and effective products is the basic regulatory responsibility of the FDA. Although its primary role is to establish standards and to review manufacturing claims, the FDA contributes to product development by providing cooperative scientific support to manufacturers particularly in the development or validation of in-process control testing. In response to the scientific challenges of regulation, the FDA has engaged in *in-vitro* and animal experimentation and epidemiologic surveillance to validate product safety or efficacy. Examples include research studies on the partitioning and inactivation of HIV-1 by Cohn-Oncley fractionation to make immune globulin [2], and a study of the efficacy of the HIV p24 antigen test for donor screening [3]. More recently, research activity has focused on virus inactivation procedures for clotting factor concentrates, the safety of IGIV made from plasma screened for anti-HIV and validation of improved screening tests for infectious diseases based on recombinant DNA-derived or synthetic antigens and possibly by gene amplification.

New products may also contribute to improved safety by reducing the need for homologous blood. Examples include autologous blood, erythropoietin and DDAVP. The Agency is also reviewing potential product claims for red cell substitutes such as hemoglobin solutions.

Summary

The US system of regulation related to transfusion medicine evolved in the context of a private industry in a free market. In response to the problems of the past, federal laws were enacted which progressively empowered the government to establish and enforce manufacturing standards for blood and blood products. Current standards apply to donor suitability, donor and product testing, manufacturing procedures (collection, processing, quarantine, labelling, storage and release), record keeping and retrieval, and quality assurance. By vigorous surveillance and enforcement, the FDA insures that all requirements are met. Consistent enforcement of regulations both maintains a uniform standard and promotes public confidence in products which are needed to save lives. FDA review and validation of new or modified products and procedures further insure that such changes will be examined in a scientific light, for the public good, prior to commercialization.

The basis of FDA regulation includes authority related to approval of establishments and products, and authority related to surveillance and enforcement. The publication of appropriate regulations is a major element in the establishment of regulatory controls, however, liberal use is made of less formal communications. The publication of guidance documents is used to facilitate compliance with regulations. Although it maintains confidentiality with manufacturers, the FDA develops its policies through a process which includes many opportunities for public comment and the advice of outside experts. The FDA evolves new standards through product reviews which are responsive to new scientific knowledge, including the results of its own basic and applied research.

References

1. Leitman SF, Klein HG, Melpolder JJ, et al. Clinical implications of positive tests for antibodies to human immunodeficiency virus type 1 in asymptomatic blood donors. N Engl J Med 1989;321:917-24.
2. Wells MA, Wittek AE, Epstein JS, et al. Inactivation and partitioning of human T-cell lymphotropic virus, type III, during ethanol fractionation of plasma. Transfusion 1986;26:210-3.
3. Alter H, Epstein JS, Swenson S, et al. Determination of the prevalence of HIV-1 p24 antigen in US blood donors: Assessment of efficacy for blood donor screening. N Engl J Med 1990;323:1312-7.

LIABILITY ARISING FROM THE ADMINISTRATION OF BLOOD AND BLOOD PRODUCTS WITHIN THE EUROPEAN ECONOMIC COMMUNITY

J.D. Evans

Introduction

Over recent years in a number of states around the world claims for compensation have been made by hemophiliacs who had been treated with blood products infected by the HIV virus. England was no exception to this and the claims, except for the clinical negligence element alleged in some cases, have been settled recently by the Government. Now, apparently, there are some hundreds of claims for compensation being prepared by English patients who allege they have been infected with hepatitis C or the HIV virus as a result of blood transfusions. In England the hemophiliacs claims were dealt with under the English Common Law. Increasingly there is going to be a European dimension to claims of this nature. One of the main trends within the Community is towards the protection of the individual, the consumer, including the patient.

On the 25th July 1985 the Council of the European Economic Community issued a Directive (85/374/EEC) concerning liability for defective products. Member states of the Community should have introduced legislation giving effect to the directive by the 25th July 1988. Not all did. In England such legislation is effective in relation to products supplied after 1st March 1988.

On the 20th December 1990, the European Commission issued a Proposal for a Council Directive on the Liability of Suppliers of Services. It is likely to be some years before this Proposal results in a Directive and before that Directive is enacted in the laws of member states. Until this happens compensation from injury arising from the diagnosis and treatment of a patient will be subject to the individual laws and rules of member states, except for the product liability dimension.

The preamble to the Product Liability Directive lists a number of reasons for it and in particular states that the existing divergencies in the laws of member states may distort competition and affect the movement of goods within the Common Market and entail a differing degree of protection of the consumer against damage caused by a defective product. Subject to the provisions of the Directives relating to pharmaceutical products (which are not the subject of this paper) and the proposed General Safety Directive, blood and blood products are dealt with as any other product and are subject to the same provisions of the Product Liability Directive. The proposed Services Liability Directive is directed more towards consumer safety than preventing distortions in trade and the explanatory memorandum makes it clear that included amongst the liabilities it is looking at is the liability of providers of health care. There are certainly no express exemptions from the Product Liability Directive for products used in health care and given the purpose of the proposed Services Liability Directive it is difficult to see health care being excluded from it.

The purpose of this paper is to examine the existing provisions on product liability and what is proposed on service liability and to consider some of the consequences that may impinge in the health care field and in particular relating to blood and blood products.

The product liability directive

The effect of this Directive can be summarised: "The PRODUCER is liable to the consumer (patient) for damage caused by a DEFECT in its PRODUCT, unless it has a DEFENCE".

The words emphasised have artificial meanings and in the context of product liability care must be taken in their use.

A PRODUCER includes: the Manufacturer; the Producer of any raw material; Anyone who by putting his name, trademark or other distinguishing feature on the product presents himself as its producer; Anyone who imports the product into the European Community; and, where the producer cannot be identified, each supplier of the product unless that supplier forms the injured person, when asked, of the identity of the person who supplied him.

There is a DEFECT in a product when it does not provide the safety which a person is entitled to expect, taking all circumstances into account. This concept of a "Defect" is of crucial importance to the Directive, but its effect is still unclear. There is the possibility of different expectations of safety in different places or at different times. And, it is implicit that not all products have to be absolutely safe. By taking all circumstances into account, it is possible that a product would be without a "Defect" to one consumer who received a prior warning of its inherent risks and would have a "Defect" for another consumer who was not warned. That a drug has a side effect does not necessarily mean that it is a Product with a "Defect".

PRODUCT certainly includes blood products, but perhaps not blood. Drafts of the Product Liability Directive expressly excluded blood from this definition, but the Directive itself does not do so. However, even were blood a "Product" it still may be outside the terms of the Directive on the grounds that there is no "Producer" of the blood.

There are a number of ways in which a DEFENCE can arise, including the development risk, or state of the art, defence which is available to a Producer if he can prove that the state of scientific and technical knowledge at the time when he put the product into circulation was not such as to enable the existence of the defect to be discovered. Member states have the option of excluding this Defence in their own legislation. The UK domestic legislation purports to express this defence in a rather wider way by importing an element of reasonableness into the Producer's state of knowledge. As it is the defence in the Directive is a narrow one; it does not refer only to the Producer's state of knowledge, but apparently to the state of knowledge generally, and the knowledge referred to is not of the defect but knowledge which should enable a defect to be discovered. Producers may find it a difficult task to succeed in this defence.

Under the Product Liability Directive there is a limitation period of three years from the date the claimant became aware, or should reasonably have become aware, of the damage, the defect and the identity of the Producer. Rights conferred by the Directive are extinguished ten years from the date on which the Producer put into circulation the actual product that caused the damage.

Under the Product Liability Directive the consumer has to prove that a defect in the product caused the damage and who the Producer was. There is no need for the consumer to prove fault, but this is not a scheme of no fault compensation. The Producer can still avoid liability by putting forward one of the defences, or by saying that although the product caused the consumer's damage, there was no defect within the meaning of that word in the Directive.

Liability of suppliers of services

The effect of the proposed Directive can be summarized: The SUPPLIER of a SERVICE shall be liable for damage caused by a FAULT committed by him in performing the service.

Again, the emphasized words have artificial meanings and care needs to be taken in using them in the context of the proposed Directive.

SUPPLIER includes a contractor if the provision of the service is subcontracted. In the UK context, this may make a Purchaser of services liable as well as the Provider.

SERVICE means any transaction carried out on a commercial basis or by way of a public service and in an independent manner, whether or not in return for payment. This definition clearly includes medical and other health care services but the proposal does not apply to public services intended to maintain public safety. There are a number of other specific exclusions, which are not relevant here.

In assessing FAULT, account is to be taken of the behaviour of the supplier of the service, who, in normal and reasonably and foreseeable conditions, shall ensure the safety which may reasonably be expected.

The Consumer has to prove the identity of the Supplier and that the Service caused the damage, but once this is done the supplier has to prove the absence of fault, if he is to defeat the claim. Within the UK, this would be a change in the burden of proof.

The Proposal includes a limitation period of three years, as under the Product Liability Directive, but the extinguishment of rights would take place after five years from the date of provision of the service.

Under the Product Liability Directive and the proposed Service Liability Directive, liability of the Producer and the Supplier respectively to an injured person cannot be excluded, but liability can be reduced or waived where the damage is caused jointly by the fault of the Producer or Supplier and the injured person. Thus, the principles of what English lawyers call contributory negligence remain.

Discussion

Neither the Product Liability Directive nor the Service Liability Directive seek to regulate the way in which compensation is calculated when there has been a breach of the provisions of either. Thus the context in which member states give effect to the Directives will vary widely. This will give rise to forum shopping, where the injured person seeks to bring his claim in the jurisdiction which will pay him most. The scope for forum shopping is clearly greatest under the Product Liability Directive, where the Producer may well be domiciled in a state different to the final supplier. It may be expected that if this practice grows within the Community, the insurance premiums in the more generous states will rise to reflect the practice. It may well be thought that this will provide a significant distortion to trade within the Community and will give rise to a proposal to approximate the laws of member states concerning the calculation of compensation for personal injury or death.

Not only may forum shopping increase, but those who may be liable under each Directive will undoubtedly be doing their best to prove that the other is liable. It is therefore unfortunate that the two very different regimes proposed for Product Liability and Services Liability do not make it easy to ascertain where the line is to be drawn between them.

Many courts in different jurisdictions have grappled with the problems caused by the supply of goods and services as part of the one package. A patient's diagnosis, care and treatment are an inter-related package and may comprise professional judgment, services from the health care professions and the provision of a wide range of products. Is one to consider the whole package a supply of a service, with the supply of the products being ancillary, or is one to separate the whole process into its constituent parts and apply the appropriate rules to each? Different conclusions have been reached in different places. In some jurisdictions the problems caused by blood and blood products have been dealt with separately, sometimes by legislation, sometimes by case law, in a way which makes their provision a service.

At the moment there does not seem to be a clear answer within the Product Liability Directive or the proposed Service Liability Directive. It will take time before uniformity is imposed in each member state and across the European Economic Community by the case law. In the short term and in the context we are talking about, any benefit for an injured person is likely to prove illusory and hard to grasp.

Unless a hospital is its own producer of blood and blood products, it should be taking steps to limit its own product liability by keeping track of its own suppliers and by not putting its own label on products unless it is absolutely necessary. It is important also to watch the terms upon which the purchase and sale of products is done. So far as the patient is concerned the product liability of the producer cannot be excluded, but there is no reason why, by means of conditions of contract and indemnities, the ultimate financial liability should not fall on one of the suppliers, including the hospital that finally supplies the product to a patient. Therefore it is important to watch where the indemnities put this ultimate financial liability, and this is so whether you are buying or selling.

On the Services Liability side, suppliers are going to have to consider how, when claims are made, within five years, they are going to be able to prove that they had not been at fault. This could be difficult in a rapidly developing area where knowledge increases significantly and good practice changes. It is probably going to be necessary to more carefully document management decisions as to standard practices to be adopted and as to changes in existing procedures. If work is sub-contracted, again it will be important to take care as to where the indemnities and the conditions of contract leave the ultimate financial liability.

Conclusions

There is clearly going to be some increased uniformity of consumers and patients rights as against both the producer and the supplier of blood and blood products.

It is still unclear whether the administration of blood and blood products to a patient during a course of hospital treatment will be treated as the supply of a product or the supply of a service.

The distinction between what is a product and what is a service is important but indistinct and the regrettable consequence may well be simply an increase in litigation with its concomitant increase in insurance premiums.

It will take time for European Economic Community case law to develop and bring greater uniformity, but further legislation will be needed from the Commission to harmonize the consequences of consumers exercising rights under these directives.

INTERNATIONAL REGULATIONS AND LEGISLATION IN TRANSFUSION MEDICINE

R.W. Beal[1], V. Boltho-Massarelli

Those who practice transfusion medicine are increasingly aware of the importance of legislation and regulation as a means of safeguarding the best aspects of their current practice. There is, as a corollary, an increased interest in, and a turning to such legislation as exists. The AIDS epidemic has not only enhanced the interest in legislation but has brought with it a flood of legislation and litigation.

The world is shrinking, and international barriers to travel and trade are falling rapidly. People, and the blood they donate, are crossing borders more often than ever before. Increasingly, there is a need for commonality and harmonization of legislation and regulation between countries to ensure the rapid transit of blood from its source to those in need.

This paper examines some of the areas in which legislation and regulation are helpful in regard to ensuring the safety of the blood supply. It then looks at the role of international agencies and organizations, principally within Europe, and their contributions to transfusion legislation. Finally, as this is part of a series on fact and fallacy, some of the potential difficulties are noted.

Legislation and transfusion

Establishment of a National Blood Transfusion Service

It is essential for the effective operation of a national blood program that it have demonstrable support from government in several critical areas of operation. This applies whether the government operates the service or where government requests an outside agency, such as a Red Cross/Red Crescent (RCRC) Society, to undertake this responsibility. Ideally, the legislation should be part of the country's overall health legislation and should be succinct, allowing for the inevitable and necessary changes dictated by current transfusion practice to be dealt with by regulation.

---

1. This paper was presented by Prof. R.W. Beal on behalf of Mrs. V. Boltho-Massarelli, Council of Europe.

Although the Council of Europe's Recommendation R(88)4 on the responsibilities of health authorities in the field of blood transfusion refers to the adoption of common regulations in the health field and coordination of all activities, it may appear to stop short of recommending formal establishment of a service by regulation or legislation. However, it makes clear the responsibilities of Health Authorities in this area in considerable detail.

Voluntary, non-remunerated donation

In a number of countries, the concept of voluntary non-remunerated blood donation is covered by legislation, which has been enacted in order to ensure the safety of the blood supply. While this is not the place to debate the pros and cons of this issue, EEC Directive 89/381 has proposed changes within Europe to ensure that this situation is regarded as the ideal.

Sale of blood and blood products

Implicit in some countries, and explicit in others, is legislation preventing the sale of blood. In this context, blood is regarded in much the same light as another body tissue, say the kidney or liver. Problems associated with traffic in body organs have once more directed attention to the undesirability of commercial sale of blood. Article 11 of the Council of Europe's Recommendation R(88)4 advocates for reasons of ethics and safety, that where blood products are imported, the countries concerned should have appropriate "legislation and practice governing the protection of donors and recipients ...".

Donor selection criteria

In some countries, criteria have been laid down, usually by regulation, concerning the suitability (or otherwise) as blood donors of certain categories of persons within the community. In years past, such criteria were the responsibility of the transfusion services to determine at a national or more often local level, according to general guidelines. With the advent of AIDS, and the recognition of potential transmission of HIV by blood and blood products, self-exclusion by donors is often covered by legislative or regulatory requirements.

Testing criteria

The recognition that blood transfusion may carry with it the risk of transmitting infection has led to the writing of legislation or regulations in many countries, requiring that blood be tested to exclude certain specific infectious diseases. Inevitably, the legislation differs from country to country, and according to the perceived prevalence and risk of a particular disease within the country concerned. As slow as some Blood Transfusion Services (BTSs) are to implement new tests, legislation tends to be slower in its response to change. Any such requirements are better dealt with under regulations which generally are easier to amend than legislation. It is also preferable that any regulations be written in non-specific terms, in order to facilitate the inevitable updating that will occur as technology advances.

Notification criteria

Some BTSs have for many years been required to notify the appropriate health authority of would-be donors confirmed as having a potentially blood-transmissible infection. The old arguments brought by BTSs that such notification was a breach of confidentiality were overcome in part by notifying the donor's medical adviser of the result, thus making this practitioner, and not the BTS, responsible for such notification. Clearly, this may have worked in a Western society for the occasional donor who tested positive for syphilis – this mechanism is inappropriate for HIV infection, and for many countries where the donor has no formal medical adviser. Increasingly, BTSs are required to notify a responsible authority, sometimes anonymously, of such positive findings.

International agencies and legislation

Of the several international agencies involved in blood transfusion, mention is made of five in relation to legislation.

The *International Society of Blood Transfusion* is the international body of transfusion professionals, and although it was the source of the 1980 Code of Ethics, it has no legislative authority. The Code of Ethics has however influenced subsequent legislation in a number of countries.

The *League of Red Cross and Red Crescent Societies* has made statements in the form of resolutions at International Conferences, General Assemblies and the like concerning important transfusion matters, but it too has no legislative impact, even in those countries where Red Cross/Crescent is directly involved in the national blood program.

The *World Health Organization*, increasingly active in the blood transfusion arena in the past decade, and particularly since the establishment of the Global Blood Safety Initiative in 1988, also has no legislative powers. Its statements, resolutions and recommendations are just that, and have no binding or legislative power.

The *Council of Europe* has promoted blood transfusion activities since the late 1950s. The competence of the Council of Europe is very wide. It covers practically all aspects of European affairs, with the exception of defence matters. Its main objectives are to defend Human Rights, maintain the European cultural identity and meet social challenges. In this context, the Council deals with topical issues; furthering human rights in the face of the challenges posed by scientific and technological progress, helping to guide the evolution of a new multiracial and multicultural society and maintaining the level of social protection.

The Council's work in the field of health enables the member states to share experiences, to compare and evaluate different approaches and to encourage the introduction of uniform health regulations and common standards of medical care. The fact that the implications of contemporary health problems are economic, technical, social and ethical means that only an organization with a pluralist and humanist tradition such as the Council of Europe is in a position to propose solutions in accordance with the principles of the Convention on Human Rights and the Social Charter. One of the oldest sectors of activity which combines all these aspects is blood transfusion.

The *first objective* in the field of blood transfusion was that of assuring the circulation of blood products within the member states in case of urgent need, i.e. natural catastrophes. This objective was realized by means of European Agreement[1]. No. 26 of 1958 on the exchange of therapeutic substances of human origin. The text included a Protocol providing common specifications for blood and blood products. This text, therefore is both the *first piece* of European legislation in Europe and the *first text* containing standards for human products.

Its impact from a practical point of view has been twofold: it has helped in a number – be it limited – of emergency situations and has generated a series of subsequent activities, including:
- two further European Agreements (Nos 39 and 84 on the Exchange of Blood Grouping Reagents and Tissue-typing Reagents respectively);
- a service activity – the European Bank of Frozen Blood of Rare Groups (located at the CLB in Amsterdam), stocking and distributing units throughout and beyond Europe;
- training activities (more than 30 events, including courses and symposia over 25 years);
- guidelines, e.g. the Guide on the Preparation, Use and Quality Assurance of Blood Components (currently in press);
- finally, but most importantly, international regulatory texts, i.e. Recommendations on a number of crucial issues.

In the 70s new studies and cooperative research were supported by the Council of Europe in order to address the issues raised by the increasing need and demand for blood products and especially plasma products. This development, in fact, generated, over a very short period of time, a complete transformation of blood transfusion in developed countries; from skilled and devoted craftsmanship it gradually became a non-profit making industry-like enterprise, requiring investments, qualified staff, rigorous quality assurance, strong management and a program of research and development.

1. A European Agreement is a binding international treaty for those states which have ratified it.

It should be stressed that if the Council of Europe continued to devote time, money and effort to this sector, it is due to the unique combination of two factors:
- the large-scale production of blood products posed a threat to the integrity of the individual in so far as being the only source for the procurement of the raw material (just as in the case of organs), exploitation through remuneration could ensue;
- the essence of the Council of Europe's vocation being the promotion of Human Rights, the integrity of the individual needed to be defended.

Two important recommendations adopted by the Committee of Ministers:
- Recommendation No. R(88)4 on Responsibilities of health authorities in the field of blood transfusion;
- Recommendation No. R(90)9 on Plasma products and European self-sufficiency
define the principles which have to be applied to this sector, and hence embedded into national legislation of member States, in order fully to respect the philosophy of the Human Rights Convention.

Recommendation R(88)4 defines five of these basic principles and develops in a series of articles the legislative measures which health authorities should take to ensure their implementation within a comprehensive transfusion service. The basic principles incorporated in R88(4) are:
- voluntary donation;
- non-remunerated donation;
- protection of donors;
- protection of recipients;
- optimal use of blood and blood products.

Recommendation R90(9) deals with a sixth principle, that of self-sufficiency.
The fifth organisation, the *European Economic Community (EEC)*, although it includes at present only 12 member states, is the one which has the strongest legislative powers in Europe. By means of "Directives"[1] it is building up a single market ensuring the free circulation of persons, goods, capital and services.
Against this background, it is clear that the EEC's interest in blood products is limited to ensuring their free circulation within its member states. Having become a contracting party to European Agreement No. 26, on the exchange of therapeutic substances of human origin, it has automatically solved the issue as concerns blood components. In the absence of a similar text for plasma

---

1. The basic difference between a Recommendation of the Council of Europe and a Directive of the EEC is that the first *recommends* that member States take the appropriate measures to attain a specific agreed objective, the second instead *requires* member states to do so within a *common given date*.

products, the EEC had to draft a specific Directive (89/381). The persistence in some European countries, despite the long-lasting efforts of the Council of Europe, of importing plasma products using remunerated plasma from non-European countries, could have easily (through marketing strategies) destabilised comprehensive and self-sufficient national blood transfusion services providing both cellular and plasma products from voluntary unpaid donations, if no reference had been made to the different origin of the products.

EEC Directive 89/381 refers to "proprietary medicinal products" and notes "special provisions for medicinal products derived from human blood or human plasma".

The Directive applies to plasma products, not to whole blood, plasma or cellular products (Article 1), and refers specifically to those products which have "... human or human plasma as a starting material ...".

The Directive goes on to stress the importance of several matters of detail, specifying the following:
– prevent transmission of infectious diseases;
– donors/donation centres identifiable;
– safety guaranteed also by importers;
– promote self-sufficiency; and finally,
proposes encouragement of voluntary unpaid donation in these words which have caused and continue to cause consternation:
"Member States shall take the necessary measures to promote Community self-sufficiency in human blood or human plasma. For this purpose, they shall encourage the voluntary unpaid donation of blood and plasma and shall take the necessary measures to develop the production and use of products derived from human blood or human plasma coming from voluntary unpaid donations. They shall notify the Commission of such measures" (Article 3, para 4).

With the rapid approach of 1993, it is clear that the ability of some countries to abide by these requirements is in question.

Many countries have many laws about many aspects of transfusion practice; one might paraphrase the Wise Man and say "of the making of laws, there is no end".

Increasingly, as was stated earlier, there is a need for commonality and harmonization of legislation and regulation between countries, both neighbouring and remote, to ensure the rapid transit of blood and blood products in emergencies. However, the prompt transit of much needed rare blood may be impeded if there is not acceptance of collection, labelling, storage, transit and customs procedures by the receiving country. The *fact* is that legislation is needed for protection of both donor and recipient; the *fallacy* is that these very rules may impede the transport of blood from one country to another when it is needed most.

The final question must be: Are these laws effective? What is the point of a law requiring blood donors to be honest in signing the donor declaration if the penalty for false or misleading information is never invoked? What is the point of a law in one of the world's most populous countries requiring all blood to be tested for hepatitis B surface antigen, when it is well known that the law is ignored in many centres?

The *fact* is that, worldwide, there is much transfusion legislation in place; the *fallacy* is in believing that this legislation is being obeyed, and is effective.

It is time to remove the blinkers, recognize the situation for the mess that it is, and do something practical about it.

DISCUSSION

T.F. Zuck, C. Dudok de Wit

T.F. Zuck (Cincinnati, OH, USA): Prof. Gevers, you talked about the use of the word commercialization several times. At least in our country it is a major issue to define what commercialization is. Does it relate to the plasma fractionation industry, does it relate to a non-for-profit blood centre that "makes money" – has excess of revenue over expense. Could you share with us your view of what a commercial enterprise in blood, blood components and fractionated blood products is?

J.K.M. Gevers (Amsterdam, NL): If we look at the blood transfusion act which was adopted in the Netherlands in 1988 and which has not yet come to full action, we have two provisions on the aspect of non-profit. The first one is the most easy and relates to the donor. It says that the donor should not be paid for giving blood. The second one says that agencies involved in collecting blood, processing it and delivering it should not make profit out of this business. I am not as well acquainted with the field of blood transfusion as many of you are, but I can see that when you talk about directly involved agencies like blood banks, it is very easy to apply that principle. However, it may become more difficult to do so, when looking further away to other organizations, industries for instance, who are using materials and processing them and then selling them for profit. As far as I know, the Dutch law does not make it impossible for instance that plasma is collected and processed, and the finished products sold, or exported to other countries. So, there is much uncertainty about what exactly the principle of non-profit making should comprise, and where commercialization starts.

U. Rossi (Legnano, I): Prof. Gevers, you said legislation is necessary in blood transfusion, but should be limited to principles and to organizational aspects which involve teamwork and mutual responsibilities. You also said that legislation on technical details and organizational work should be avoided, because of course it is dated already when it comes out. It is difficult to change, the procedures are long, and politicians tend to forget to involve clinicians. But in many countries, Italy first of all I think, politicians like to emit decrees and to intervene very heavily in our field. As Dr. Goldfinger said, we are the only one medical specialty where this happens, even anesthesists are more free. I believe that some European or international organization should be concerned about this legislation, which is obstructing progress and causing frustration. Such an organization should emit guidelines to legislators stating which are the principles, that should be covered possibly by legislation in every country, but also set the limit by stating clearly that it is unproper for governments to legislate on scientific, technical and professional aspects, which should be better left to directives from national or international societies, scientific bodies and so on.

J.K.M. Gevers: I think it is difficult of course to stop national legislators from doing what they want to do. For instance, there are directives that give a certain basic level of protection; they say that countries must make legislation which translates the results, the end-goal into national law. However, even the EEC does not interfere with the prerogative of nations to decide how exactly they want to incorporate the basic rules established at EEC level in their national laws. I think that you are quite right if you say that very detailed regulations may be obstructive rather than helpful, however this does not exclusively relate to blood transfusion. For instance, in the Netherlands there are complaints, and rightly so, about too intensive and too detailed regulation of the organization and the finance of health care. In this field we are trying to move a little bit more to the model of indirect legislation. If we look for international guidance on this point, I think the recommendation of the Council of Europe number 88/4 is a very good example of exactly the type of guidelines you are looking for: General recommendations which national authorities can follow in developing law, e.g. transfusion law.

C.F. Högman: According to some information I recently got, as much as 63% of the plasma products in the world are produced in the for-profit sector. This of course may create some problems, because if we now want to go for voluntary blood donation and not-for-profit fractionation there is quite a gap to fill. If you have a free market like we have in Sweden, then there will be some problems when you suddenly want to fulfil the goal of national self-sufficiency. The customers might not like to deal with a monopoly situation, which you may end-up to if you want to supply exclusively with plasma from the country itself. The only solution that we have found for this problem in order to achieve the different goals is to make contracts with different fractionators, in order to fractionate the plasma from the own country in for-profit companies. This allows our customers to use the products they want to buy. I wonder if you have any comments on this rather intriguing question.

J.K.M. Gevers: I would basically like to refer back to what I said in response of the first question. Maybe Dr. Beal will be more able than I am to react to this specific point.

R.W. Beal (Geneva, CH): I do not think that I could give Dr. Högman the answer that he looks for, but I think that what he has done is to identify the conundrum which directive 89/381 poses for the majority of countries in Europe: The question of self-sufficiency is in fact a theoretical one. It may be an ideal goal, but is certainly not attainable even by a country as well-developed in its transfusion services as yours.

T.F. Zuck: There is a model of course, the Canadian system in which to be self-sufficient contract-fractionation is done for plasma through Cutter. The finished products are returned back into the Canadian Red Cross system. So, there are models that perhaps will be useful.

J.S. Epstein (Bethesda, MD, USA): The question to be addressed is whether product manufacturing on a "for-profit" basis using collections from paid donors is any longer a threat to safety. We are in a new era in terms of virus inactivation technology. We are almost at the point where all of the plasma derivatives are virologically safe, because they have been specifically virally inactivated. That should be a reason to rethink our willingness to accept the paid supplier of the raw material.

F. Peetoom: I have two issues; one has to do with an observation that was just made about the increased perfection if you will of manufacturing through safety testing. I just wondered if you would go so far as to say that paid whole blood might be reintroducible given the current status of testing. We do not have it totally under control, but let us say within the foreseeable future you might see that all viruses we know of and are important to us can be tested for. Does that mean that paid donors versus volunteer donors becomes less of an issue? Then, I have a question as to who should control, or what organization should regulate the role of the physician who prescribes blood, correctly or incorrectly, as well as the liabilities that come from that practice. Who should regulate and supervise the informed consent process to make sure that the patient knows the options between homologous blood, autologous donations, blood salvage, so that the patient is given the opportunity to participate in the decisions based on information provided. This process is deficient; where does this point of the chain of safety and resulting liabilities rest and who should control it?

J.S. Epstein: The question is whether current screening is so adequate that we could consider paid donations of whole blood. I think not. We have seen a lot of improvement in donor selection using medical histories, self-deferral etc. and also testing for various infectious disease markers. However, these processes by their nature are incomplete. We know that there is still a transfusion risk for essentially all of the infectious diseases for which we screen. This risk still remains even with the marker negative volunteer donation. We suspect that paid donors might have higher prevalency rates for these infectious conditions and also higher incidence rates associated with infectious, but marker negative, collections. So, I think, until there is viral inactivation of whole blood or cellular components of blood, that it is premature to turn the clock back and reconsider the paid donor of whole blood.

J.D. Evans (Sheffield, UK): I am quite sure that judges and juries are not the ones who should be checking up or looking after the actions of doctors. In the UK at the moment there is a trend which is really not very nice: People, who are injured as the result of the acts of others, have a tendency to use the courts to seek vengeance. Doctors who have made a bad error are even now standing trial in the UK for manslaughter. I think this is a very bad thing. The profession should be careful to regulate itself, because you know the factors that have to be taken into account. I do not think judges and juries or any outside body are the ones who can properly do that in a way that in the long term safeguards patients' care and the interests of patients.

R.W. Beal: If I can just respond briefly to that second question, I think Dr. Peetoom has put his finger on a fifth paper that should have been delivered this morning; I think the area that you talked about is not one that is subject to control or regulation. I find myself a little in disagreement with Dr. Goldfinger: He says that no other branch of the profession is regulated like ours. I am sure the pharmaceutical manufacturers would consider that FDA and many of our regulatory agencies take a marked interest in people who prescribe products. I think in this context and certainly in the view of the European legislation, blood is seen as a medicinal product. The way the blood is handled clinically is not regulated and that is something that you quite properly identified as a point we need to think further about.

J.D. Cash: I just like to return again to the point that Dr. Epstein made: Are we reaching the point when our virus inactivation procedures in the large scale pool fractionation process are such that the notion that the paid donor is less safer than the unpaid donor is no longer really significant. I thought that was the point Dr. Epstein was trying to make or at least trigger some debate. In the context of the question in relation to whole blood, I strongly support his conclusions. The question that he has posed to use is an important one and it is worth trying to address. It is my view that it is probable if we had the information, and this information is now emerging in certain countries, that key to answering this question will come from looking at the viral contamination in aliquots from the pool of plasma that is to go forward to fractionation. When this information is available we may discover that in some countries the contaminating level of virus in their starting pools is higher from their unpaid local donors than from certain sources of paid donors. I think this data will emerge over the next couple of years. However excellent we think our viral inactivation procedures are, they are inevitably dependant on the starting load of viral contamination. Thus, for some countries the notion of getting large scale fractionation products in the future from paid donor plasma may in the event be preferable in terms of safety, provided there is a guarantee of system which ensures that this quality differential is sustained.

M. Rustam (Jakarta, IND): Dr. Epstein, do you have any regulation of the plasma product derived from human placenta? In our country plasma product derived from human placenta produced in France is marketed commercially. But I heard this product cannot be used in France. It is only destined for export.

J.S. Epstein: In the United States we are certainly aware that many blood products can be derived from placental tissue and we are aware specifically of Institut Merieux's program. Nevertheless, we have not found it possible to approve placental derived products mainly on the basis that it is impossible to screen the donors. Usually the manner in which the placentas are derived erases all history of the collection. Neither retrieval of donor information nor product testing is feasible. For the reason explained earlier we do not think that material collected from an arbitrary source will yield a completely safe product solely because of the manufacturing procedure. Rather, we still believe that donor selection and donor testing are significant safeguards which place limits on the infectious burden in the source material. Therefore, we have not approved any placental derived products. However, I do think that this position is open to scientific argument for certain products.

R. Kay (Gibraltar): I run the smallest blood bank in the world in Gibraltar. I think, we all agree that blood transfusion services should be founded on voluntary non-paid donors and that the organization should be non-profit making. Does the panel think, because of the threats of litigation, which are costing the patient more and more, increasing the price of the products more and more, that the lawyers who take these things to court should be non-profit making too and that they should do it voluntary.

C.Th. Smit Sibinga: It is quite obvious from the different presentations that governments should be heavily involved in the legislative and regulatory mechanisms. That is a fact as such, but the fiction is in the implementation. Prof. Gevers stated that the law should not be too restrictive and should not be too exhaustive in its regulations, but immediately following that Dr. Epstein told us that if you want to regulate, you have to have a very strict system of guidelines and standards. Otherwise there is no way of really coming to a regulation and an inspection. That seems to be somewhat controversial.

J.K.M. Gevers: Well, I do not see so much contradiction. At least it refers also to the fact that apart from regulations which have direct legal force, there are guidelines, memoranda etc. which are much more flexible and can be more easily brought up to date. So, that fits quite well into the approach, which I have called the indirect approach to legislation and which makes more room for self-regulation to some extent and for self-inspection.

C.Th. Smit Sibinga: I agree on that. However, the point is that if we come to legislation and set an act or a law controlling more or less all the different items related to blood transfusion, the protection of the donor, the recipient, the various aspects of the production, that act as such will only have an impact in reality, when there is a control mechanism to see whether we really follow what has been outlined. That means that the regulatory authorities, who are there to execute and to control the law, should have something in their hands to follow for inspection or audit, to see whether one really complies with the regulations. It is noticeable, that there are a number of countries now that do have a law, specifically on transfusion, but not a mechanisms to control whether the practice complies with the legislation. There are countries, where outside the mechanism of legislation a control mechanism within the professional group of workers is instituted – the AABB is a very good example. The United States do have both mechanisms; there is an FDA control and there is a professional institute coming to audit, accredit and certify the practice of transfusion medicine.

T.F. Zuck: Mr. Evans, I understand the law has been changed at least at the EEC level from saying that the burden of proof is on the plaintiff to prove that the blood centre did something wrong or negligent to now require the blood centre to proof that everything was done perfectly. This appears to me to be a major change in how we keep records. The specific question is, should the blood centres now have some kind of audit procedure, not only to say that scientifically the components were safe and the tests were done well, but also that they are found perfect as examined in a legal forum in order to survive?

J.D. Evans: Yes, you should have some audit process that is in writing and that will survive for the five or ten years it is needed to keep you out of any trouble with the courts. It is going to be important for you to be able to show that you treated the patient without fault on your part. Now, fault is not something that is absolute; it is something that is going to be judged depending on the state of knowledge, depending on the acceptable practice, depending on the cost of what you can do, the public policy aspects of how much cost one can allocate to health care. All these factors are going to be considered, but you must be in the position to show that you have taken into account all the relevant factors and reached some recent decision as to the process and the practice that you followed. Audit is one way to do that and one should keep the records of it. Audit is not something to be frightened of for other people looking at it. Audit is something that you can use as a shield. You should bear it in mind and use it as a shield.

D.B.L. McClelland: Mr. Evans, in relation to the 85 directive, would you advise us as producers, that we should now be taking steps to inform all potential transfusion recipients of the potential risks about transfusion and also where appropriate of the possibilities that might be open to receive an alternative treatment such as a predeposit autologous transfusion?

J.D. Evans: The more the patient knows about the risks of treatment, the less risk you have of a claim. this area in the UK at the moment is not a high-risk area for claims. So, the short answer to the question is no, I do not think you need to do that. I do not think you need to inform the patient of these sorts of risks and the alternatives that the patient could be dealt with. However, the more information the patient has, the better. The more you talk to the patient, the less risk there is of claims. So, in that respect it is certainly worthwhile thinking and planning down the route of informing the patient more and more.

J.K.M. Gevers: A brief comment on the presentation of Mr. Evans. I was a bit puzzled by the fact that you said that there is so much uncertainty about basic concepts in the EC directive of 1985 concerning product and producer in relation to blood transfusion. We have implemented also in the Netherlands that EC directive a little later than you have done in England, but there was consensus in our parliament that blood is a product in the sense of the EC directive. In the sense of the national law adopted to that directive in the normal situation, a blood bank should be considered as a producer and should be liable therefore as a producer.

B.T. Teague: Prof. Beal, you listed the first principle as a volunteer donor and the second as a non-remunerated donor. I would like to understand the difference between those two terms. The second question is that you indicated legislation had been introduced to prevent the sale of blood. Could you define the sale of blood?

R.W. Beal: To answer the first question: The difference between voluntary and non-remunerated. Companies in the plasma industry make the point that their donors give voluntarily. In other words they are not coerced, there is no compulsion brought on the person and that it is the act of volunteering to do so. Non-remunerated simply means no cash and nothing that can be redeemed for cash. In other words no money changes hands, nor goods that can be translated into money. So, I think the two of them are separated. The problems I think come into translation here, because as the French speakers in the audience will know, neither the word voluntary nor non-remunerated comes through very well in French. They have much better words, which translated into English mean benevolent and altruistic. Benevolent has a totally different meaning in English from its French meaning, which is most appropriate to what we talk about as voluntary non-remunerated blood donation. The word altruism is in the English language, but most people who give blood do not know what it means. So, we do have a problem with semantics; I agree with you.

Regarding the sale of blood, this was in fact a reference to a person offering his blood for sale in the same way as there is legislation preventing people offering organs for sale. It is quite an old act; it is mostly taken up in more recent times in acts dealing with transplantation and preventing the sale of organs, including blood.

B.T. Teague: Just as a clarification, so that relates to the donor selling rather than the producer selling to a hospital.

R.W. Beal: Yes.

III. EDUCATIONAL ASPECTS

STANDARDS, INSPECTION AND ACCREDITATION MECHANISMS IN TRANSFUSION MEDICINE

C.Th. Smit Sibinga, P.C. Das

Introduction

Like in any other profession, practice in medicine should be based on well defined criteria. These criteria should relate to the benefit and safety of the patient and the personnel involved, the principle adagium being the "primum est non nocere".

However, criteria should not hamper personal responsibility of the medical practitioner towards each individual patient. Too restrictive and regulatory criteria may have a negative effect on the quality of medical practice towards the individual patient. In this respect the quality of practice does not exclusively depend on the individual practitioner, but intimately relates to:
- the code of practice; and
- the specifically defined criteria of practice or standards, their implementation and audit.

In any medical discipline it is the responsibility of the group of professionals to safeguard the quality and standard of practice in their specific field by setting and accepting a code of practice and defining and updating the criteria and standards of practice according to the state of the art and the ongoing developments.

As the field of transfusion medicine deals with that part of the health care system which undertakes the appropriate provision and use of human blood resources, whether whole blood, plasma or cells, the group of professionals is explicitly multi-disciplinary: Medical, pharmaceutical, biochemical, socio-medical. If we assume that transfusion practice is that collective action which links the blood donor with the patient, then it follows that transfusion medicine occupies those areas in which it is deemed important or even essential that a medical practitioner contributes to this bridging process.

Audit or inspection

To warrant the quality of "Good Medical Practice" audit should be accepted as a useful and adequate means of review and control. A regularly used mechanism of audit is inspection through qualified peer review. Such a mechanism could provide a system of independence and objectivity needed to support and sustain the confidence in and fundamental attitude to the principle of quality assurance and the related reality of "Good Medical Practice".

The mechanism of peer review can be achieved through trained and qualified inspectors, selected on the basis of defined criteria from the field of transfusion practice. Inspectors in action just follow the standards; they check whether the standards are practised, and if not ask for explanation as alternative methods and approaches may allow equally safe practice.

For audit purposes the standards should be translated into an inspection report form (IRF), which serves as a guide for the inspection and just needs to be filled in and completed by the inspector. The inspection report form could provide several categories of information, such as statistical and organizational information, informative questions, questions which harbour an advisory suggestion and the norms stipulated in the standards per se. An affirmative answer to the latter and ultimate audit questions confirm "Good Medical Practice", where a negative answer in principle reflects a deviation from the standards and therefore should be interpreted as a deficiency which needs corrective action. Informative questions could provide valuable information that may lead to improvement of the practice, where the advisory suggestions could be used for the next upgrading of the standards.

To adequately and correctly use the IRF, the inspector should be imbued with the ultimate purpose of audit or inspection: To aid in developing and maintaining procedures that will provide safe and effective donor-to-patient practice, as well as safe environment for personnel.

Standards

The mechanisms to warrant "Good Medical Practice" in any discipline are complex and relate to a large extent to attitude and mentality of all personnel involved. Here education is the key-concept to a clear and simple explanation of what is to be done. The nucleus of the explanatory process to any individual worker should be the definition of standards of practice, accepted in consensus and based on clearly defined expertise and job descriptions. This will provide a means for adequate and competent staffing.

As medicine develops through science, new developments are tested in medical practice, validated or rejected to the benefit of patient care and safety. Subsequently they are implemented, become routine and thus require reproducibility to allow consequently standard of practice. Therefore, standards have to be in writing and regularly updated and adapted to the new developments as to secure the quality of practice. They are meant to be helpful rather than restrictive. The requirements described should be simple, clear and practical, and should serve as the minimum acceptable standard of practice. The most important aspect of standards is not in the technical details and their implementation, but in the reflection in human attitude and mentality: The sincere and professional desire to warrant the quality of "Good Medical Practice".

Once standards have been accepted in consensus by the groups of professionals, they should be implemented. The process of implementation not only includes the technical and administrative aspects, but more explicitly the explanation and motivation of the aims and purposes of the implementation to all personnel involved. This process of mental training is the ultimate fundament for a successful mechanism of quality assurance.

Inspectors

Inspectors should be selected from the field of transfusion practice on well defined criteria. They should have substantial experience in the field of transfusion medicine, preferably at senior staff level.

Inspectors should be trained and continuously educated both through informative courses and practical exercises. They should know the standards, and their explanation. They should be flexible and understanding, and should know how to control conflicts. An audit or inspection is almost always perceived as intrusive and sometimes even offensive. Therefore the inspector should know that there is a potential for controversies and conflicts. Handling and controlling such situations is probably the most difficult part of the job, as the purpose is supportive rather than criticizing. To avoid such controversies and conflictuous situations, inspectors should never inspect on mutual grounds and avoid debate. The attitude should be helpful and supportive, with an obvious willingness to assist in solving problems.

Following the actual audit or inspection, the inspector should not leave the facility before having reviewed the immediate inspection results with the responsible staff, in order to allow necessary supplementary information to be given and to discuss possible options and guidance for corrective action.

Accreditation

Following the inspection and completion of the IRF, a list of deficiencies, quiries and recommendations for corrective action is provided. The inspected facility should be given ample opportunity to organize and implement appropriate corrective action, which should be reported back in writing. Once it has been shown that the facility meets or even exceeds the standards, representing the accepted performance guidelines, the procedure should result in accreditation for a given period of time. Accreditation should be provided through a signed and dated certificate (Figure 1).

American Association of Blood Banks

Herewith certifies that

Red Cross Bloodbank Groningen-Drenthe

having been examined by the American Association of Blood Banks, has been found to meet the administrative and technical standards of this organization and therefore this blood bank is granted this

CERTIFICATION OF ACCREDITATION

In Witness Whereof the undersigned officers, being duly authorized, have caused this Certificate to be issued and the Corporate Seal of this Association to be affixed hereon this the

28 th day of February 1984

This Certificate expires

December 1985

unless extended in accordance with approved AABB Inspection and Accreditation Procedures and Policies.

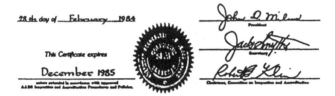

Figure 1. Certificate of accreditation of the American Association of Blood Banks.

Organization of an inspection mechanism

It is advisable that in a country the group of professionals in Transfusion Medicine develops and implements an audit or inspection mechanism to warrant "Good Blood Banking and Transfusion Practice". Such a mechanism could be complemented by a Health Authority inspection system, which primarily aims at protection of the public health against malpractice and insubordination to the law; safety and efficacy are key-concepts.

As a model a national inspection and accreditation system could be developed and organized through a national inspection and accreditation committee. To prevent cross-inspections on mutual grounds, it is advisable to divide the country into arbitrary regions of equal size and number of blood banks. Each region could then be represented in parity in the committee, and the committee be chaired by a national coordinator of the national inspection and accreditation system. In each region one of the representatives could serve on a rotating basis as a region coordinator, organizing and supervising the inspections. Regional inspectors can then be selected on the defined criteria from the senior staff of the facilities in the region. They are assigned inspection in a neighbouring region, where no two regions should cross-inspect each other (Figure 2).

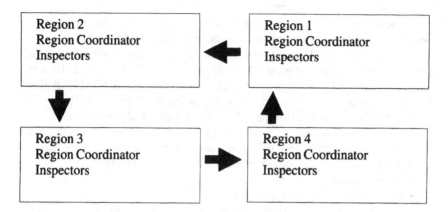

Figure 2. The region coordinators and inspectors from the regions 1, 2, 3 and 4 co-ordinate and execute the inspections in the assigned blood banks in the regions 2, 3, 4 and 1, respectively.

The procedures should be precisely and accurately outlined and documented to avoid conflict and the committee should on regular terms report back to the group of professionals in order to maintain confidence and to sustain the purpose and principles of the system: The provision of safe and effective donor-to-patient practice as well as safe environment for personnel in Transfusion Medicine.

Facts and fictions

Fact is that in transfusion medicine standards have been developed and implemented in only a limited number of countries. However, the completion of the system of national quality assurance with a mechanism of inspection and accreditation as a matter of fact is still largely fictitious.

By far the most experience is gathered and compiled by the American Association of Blood Banks. In 1957 the American Association of Blood Banks introduced a first trial edition of Standards for Accreditation of a Blood Transfusion Service [1], and implemented a system of inspection and accreditation on a national basis. The Standards are currently in their 14th edition and a 15th edition is under development.

In 1985 the Netherlands Blood Transfusion Society published the first edition of the Dutch Standards for Blood Banks, established in close cooperation with the State Control Laboratory of the Ministry of Health.

In 1989 the Federation of Dutch Red Cross Blood Banks instituted a National Inspection and Accreditation Program with a National Inspection and Accreditation Policy Committee. The fourth edition of the Dutch Standards for Blood Banks of 1990 served as the first edition which in consensus was implemented in transfusion practice; February 1991 the program started with inspection and accreditation of the first Dutch Red Cross Blood Bank.

There are at present a few more countries where such a mechanism has been instituted or is currently being developed and/or implemented.

In 1978 the World Health Organization published the first edition of the Requirements for the Collection, Processing and Quality Control of Human Blood and Blood Products in their Technical Report Series 626 [2]. A first update was published in 1989 in the Technical Report Series 786 [3].

In 1986 the Council of Europe in Strasbourg published a recommendation on Quality Control in Blood Transfusion Services [4], and is currently developing further documents. Both WHO and Council of Europe recommendations are to be conceived as an important and factual aid to come to:
– National Standards,
– mechanisms of audit or inspection,
to establish safe and sustainable practice in transfusion medicine and equivalence of performance guidelines in the respective countries.

However regretful, reality is that the respective groups of authors of both the WHO and the Council of Europe recommendations have to be classified as expert fictionists.

References

1. Standards American Association of Blood Banks, trial edition, Phoenix, AZ, 1957.
2. WHO Expert Committee on Biological Standardization. Technical Report Series 626, World Health Organization, Geneva, 1978.
3. WHO Expert Committee on Biological Standardization. Technical Report Series 786, World Health Organization, Geneva, 1989.
4. Quality control in blood transfusion services. Council of Europe, Strasbourg, 1986.

TRAINING IN TRANSFUSION MEDICINE: PROGRAMS AND MECHANISMS

W.N. Gibbs

The World Health Organization (WHO) has promoted training of health care professionals working in blood transfusion services (BTSs) for more than 20 years. Thus, it has promoted the establishment and development of local programs by providing technical assistance and by facilitating the provision of the necessary resources. This has been supplemented by the organization of training courses and production of training documents and other training materials. Table 1 lists some of the characteristics of the training courses organized by the responsible unit at WHO Headquarters between 1978 and 1990 in which serological techniques, storage of blood and blood products, quality assurance and management have been the most prominent topics. It should be pointed out that similar training courses have also been organized by the Regional Offices and also at the country level.

These efforts in training have intensified since the launch of the global Blood Safety Initiative (GBSI) in May 1988. This is a cooperative endeavour to support the development of safe and effective BTSs in all countries, and training is one of the strategies being followed to achieve this objective. The

Table 1. Short courses on blood transfusion services organized by WHO/HQ (1975-1990).

Year/country	Topic		No. countries
1978/Burundi	organization		19
1979/Kenya	general		13
1981/China	general		1
1983/Hungary	management		14
1983/Senegal	management		10
1985/Zambia	development	of BTSs at peripheral level	1
1987/Nepal	development	of BTSs at peripheral level	2
1988/Sudan	development	of BTSs at peripheral level	6
1988/Tanzania	development	of BTSs at peripheral level	5
1989/Zaire	development	of BTSs at peripheral level	9
1990/Malawi	development	of BTSs at peripheral level	5

GBSI Secretariat believes that this should encompass all of the activities in blood transfusion practice from blood donor motivation to the transfusion of blood and blood products, and that there should be provision for training of all of the health care professionals involved.

Three main areas of blood transfusion practice can be clearly identified:
- blood donor motivation, recruitment, selection and retention;
- processing of blood, including collection, testing, preparation of products, storage and distribution;
- appropriate use of blood and blood products.

Underpinning all of these is management, which is an important component of each of the three areas listed above. It should be included to a varying extent in the curriculum of the people being trained, depending on their level of expertise and responsibility.

GBSI global training plan

The GBSI Secretariat global training plan, which was drawn up during an informal consultation in November 1989 [1], takes into account the wide variation in background and experience of staff working in BTSs. The professional staff may include medical practitioners, blood donor motivators and organizers, technical staff, scientists, nurses and managers, and they are supported by secretaries and ancillary staff. The categories of staff in any BTS will depend upon the customs within the country and the level of its activity, and this list does not imply that all of the categories of staff will be required everywhere.

Principles of training

During this consultation the following principles of training were enunciated:
- Training should be carried out at the local level wherever this is practicable.
- Government commitment is necessary, including involvement in the design of training programs, support of the trainees during their training and the subsequent provision of posts in order to make a career structure possible.
- The objective, scope and design of training programs should take into account the evolving nature of transfusion medicine, and the varying circumstances in different countries.
- When certificates or diplomas are issued they should be relevant to the requirements of the country in terms of personnel structure and professional standards.
- Trainees and courses must be monitored and evaluated.

Training programs and methods

The aim of all training is to give the trainees the opportunity to acquire the necessary knowledge, skills and attitude so that they will function competently in relation to their post description. The GBSI global training plan includes: defining training needs; promotion of apprentice-type training programs; facilitating the organization of training courses; and preparing training materials.

Defining training needs

A survey carried out recently by the GBSI Secretariat demonstrated that most countries have not determined their training needs – neither the numbers and categories of staff to be trained, nor the content of the training programs or courses. As has been pointed out above, the numbers and categories of staff to be trained will vary according to the customs in the country and the activity of the BTS. an informal consultation held in April 1991 [2] provided guidelines to determine these.

The course or program content will be determined by the training objectives. The latter are determined in turn by the postdescription for each category of staff. The consultation suggested the use of a task-oriented grid system to

Table 2. Example of the use of a grid system to determine training objectives.

Tasks	Medical pract.	Technical staff	Nurses	Blood donor organizers
Blood donors:				
motivation	2*	3	2	1
recruitment	2	3	2	1
selection	2	3	2	1
retention	2	3	2	1
Blood processing:				
collection	2	2	1	3
testing	2	1	3	3
storage	1	1	3	3
product preparation	1	1	3	3
distribution	1	1	3	3
Appropriate use of blood:	1	2	2	3
Management:				
financial	1	2	3	3
personnel	1	2	3	3
quality assurance	1	1	2	3
logistics	1	2	3	3

* Numbers refer to levels of responsibility (see text).

help in drawing up course objectives based on the activities of each category of staff.

An application of this system is illustrated in Table 2 for a country in which the professional staff consists of medical practitioner(s), technical staff, nurses and blood donor organizer(s). The numbers in the table refer to levels of responsibility for performing activities and related tasks: level "1" indicates the major responsibility; level "2" indicates a supporting role; and level "3" indicates responsibility common to all professional staff in the BTS, regardless of their roles.

Thus, in this example the medical practitioner's activities will be primarily in management, clinical interaction (appropriate use of blood) and some aspects of blood processing (storage, product preparation and distribution). These aspects of processing are shared with the technical staff who are, in addition, primarily responsible for laboratory testing. Nurses carry the major responsibility for collecting blood; and blood donor organizers for motivating, recruiting, selecting and retaining donors.

Training objectives are formulated from the activities set out in Table 2. Training curricula and programs are drawn up from these objectives and activities, and from more detailed tasks based on the latter, with appropriate weighting for details of the topics to be covered and the length of time to be spent on each. Ideally, the training program should include an introduction covering the four main areas of blood transfusion practice for all members of staff together. This would be followed by more detailed aspects, as appropriate, for each category of staff. However, there should be interaction between the different categories of BTS during training whenever possible, and also between trainees in transfusion medicine and those in related disciplines, such as laboratory medicine, hematology and immunology.

Programs and courses

Apprentice-type training programs provide an excellent opportunity for development of knowledge, skills and attitude, particularly since they include various methods of continuing education. The main disadvantage from the point of view of many developing countries is the relatively large amount of resources necessary, so that facilities are not as widely available as they should be. On the other hand, many countries cannot afford to send their nationals abroad for the long periods of time required for this type of training and, in some cases, the training acquired abroad is inappropriate. GBSI is developing criteria for the guidance of national authorities for establishing or developing national training institutions. These criteria can also be used for the recognition of regional training centres, and for guidance in selection of training centres farther afield. GBSI will also help to identify and mobilize resources, and provide technical advice and support.

Training courses have been arbitrarily divided into short-term (two to four weeks) and long-term (three to six months). The main role of GBSI is to identify needs globally to mobilize resources and, in some cases, to organize the courses. Members of the GBSI Secretariat have also participated as faculty in some of these courses.

The short-term courses are designed to provide the basic knowledge and skills in transfusion medicine; to train tutors; or to provide updates on a variety of topics in which weaknesses have been identified. The latter include: donor motivation, recruitment, selection and care; management; equipment; reagent production; quality assurance in transfusion medicine; techniques for screening for infectious agents; the appropriate use of blood; and autologous transfusion.

Long-term courses cover aspects of transfusion medicine deemed to be necessary for the trainees based on the assessment of training needs. They consist of classroom training (theory and practice) and in-service training, thus providing an opportunity for more comprehensive training than is possible with the short-term courses but without most of the disadvantages already outlined for the apprentice-type training programs. A major problem is that it is very difficult to find the resources for this type of training course: it has been possible to launch only one course so far.

Production of training materials

Production of training materials has been undertaken by the GBSI to supplement the courses mentioned above and to be adapted by health care workers to the needs of their countries. Seven manuals or consensus statements are in draft form or in press [see 3-8], some of them replacing documents which have become obsolete. Videotapes have also been produced. The justification for producing these materials is that they are more affordable than most of those produced commercially, and they take into account the limited resources of developing countries without compromising standards.

More recently, the GBSI has been developing *distance learning materials* to be used particularly in those countries where a shortage of trained staff makes it difficult for them to attend courses elsewhere. Modules are being developed at two levels: for training tutors; and for training at a basic level. Because they involve self-learning in the trainees' environment, an essential corollary is the provision of the basic infrastructure so that, for example, the requisite practical work can be undertaken.

Monitoring and evaluation (see Table 3)

Many training courses and programs are organized globally, but few are adequately evaluated. It is relatively easy to devise indicators for monitoring the planning and organization of training programs and courses.

Table 3. Monitoring and evaluation.

Programs and courses:
immediate
- organization and planning
- relevance
- faculty

long-term
- effectiveness and impact

Trainees:
- acquisition of knowledge, skills
- performance

This includes information available to the organizers and faculty, and feedback from the trainees. The trainees will also provide information about the relevance of the course or program to their needs and the performance of the faculty. Assessment of the trainees should include comparison of their performance at (or before) the start and at the end of the program or course, combined with continuing assessment. The latter is particularly valuable for assessing the development of skills.

It is much more difficult to assess the effectiveness and impact of training. Questions must be devised so that the assessment can be carried out objectively and in a standardized way, but without too much disruption for the people who were trained or for their supervisors. It is particularly difficult to get the cooperation of the participants and their supervisors when they are from more than one country. A priority and challenge for GBSI is to devise a scheme to resolve this problem.

Acknowledgments

This acknowledges the help of several experts in drawing up the GBSI global training plan in transfusion medicine. I thank my colleagues in the GBSI Secretariat for giving me the opportunity to present the information in this paper on their behalf.

References

1. World Health Organization. Report on informal consultation on training in transfusion medicine. November 1989, Appendix 1: GBSI global training plan in transfusion medicine.
2. World Health Organization. Report on informal consultation on assessment of training needs in transfusion medicine. April 1991 (in preparation).
3. World Health Organization. Global blood safety initiative. Use of plasma substitutes and plasma in developing countries. WHO/LAB/89.9.

4. World Health Organization. Global blood safety initiative. Autologous transfusion in developing countries. WHO/LBS/91.2.
5. World Health Organization. Global blood safety initiative. The preparation of cryo-precipitate (videotape).
6. World Health Organization. Global blood safety initiative. Blood donors for safe blood transfusion: Facing the AIDS challenge (in preparation).
7. World Health Organization. Global blood safety initiative. Manual on blood group serology and preparation of blood grouping reagents (in preparation).
8. World Health Organization. Global blood safety initiative. Guidelines for a quality assurance programme for blood transfusion services (in preparation).

THE NEED FOR CONTINUOUS EDUCATION AND PERFORMANCE APPRAISAL

S.J. Urbaniak

As professionals, physicians are expected to self-regulate, to maintain standards and assess fitness to practice in a given specialty. The law only sets basic minimum standards (medical degree) to protect the public from non-doctors, and only acts *post facto* in cases of criminal negligence, malpractice etc. It is up to the profession to set the highest standards from within if unduly restrictive or punitive regulations are not to be imposed. In the UK, the General Medical Council is responsible for maintaining the medical register; it is essential to be on the register to practice legally as a doctor, and the ultimate sanction is to be "struck off". Unfortunately it only requires a few well publicized incidents for public perception of medical competence to be damaged, and there is a need for the profession to be *seen* to be acting responsibly in setting standards. Whilst it is undeniable that there is a need for all doctors to remain proficient and up-to-date, the means by which this can be achieved is not straightforward.

Although in the eyes of the law any medically qualified person can undertake any medical procedure (and will only intervene if something goes wrong) the restriction of practice to an area where the individual is properly and adequately trained has been a topic of medical debate for centuries. Fierce argument about who was fit to practice what originated between physicians and surgeons, and continues to the present day between hematologists, transfusionists and others. The right to define a specialty, set standards, conduct examinations, and allow entry to a specialty has been jealously guarded by existing interests, but in an age where the advance of medicine scientifically and technically has been spectacular, subspecialisation has become necessary to practice at the highest level. This in turn generates problems of assessment of competence for entry to a specialist register, and once on the register, keeping up to date with progress in the specialty. In the UK, the former is reasonably well defined; the latter is not.

In the case of specialists (consultants), a very high level of practical and theoretical expertise is demanded in a relatively limited area compared to primary care GPs, and consultants do not deal directly with the public but only on referral from GPs and other consultants. To an extent there is a degree of protection of the public from consultants who might be tempted to stray from their primary specialty, and a "poor performer" will get fewer referrals, but clearly in the NHS where salaries are fixed there is a need for a more structured approach to assessing and maintaining professional expertise.

Trainees

The educational and training program which a trainee specialist should follow is, in principle, clearly defined and the job description includes continuous education and continued progress as a requirement (Figure 1). In the UK the job description is not a central element to defining training needs or responsibilities, and there is no formal mechanisms of performance appraisal. What we have is a formal framework which is applied informally in that there is a minimum of paperwork, there is no requirement to provide proof of having carried out a given number of procedures etc. nor to have certification of having achieved a particular standard in carrying out various specialist tasks. The current system is summarised below.

Scottish Health Service Common Services Agency

Division:	Scottish National Blood Transfusion Service
Title of post:	Senior Registrar
Grade:	Senior Registrar (whole time)
Responsible to:	Regional Director
Location:	– Base: [ ] Regional Transfusion Centre
	– Rotation to another SNBTS Centre for approximately one year

Duties and responsibilities
1. Full information about the functions of the Department and the SNBTS Medical Training Program are attached.
2. The appointee will be required to undertake a full program of training in transfusion medicine.
3. The appointee will take a full part in the clinical and laboratory duties shared by the centre's medical staff, including on-call duties and participation in blood donation and plasmapheresis sessions and will act as secretary to the Regional Centre's Medical Audit Committee.
4. The appointee will be encouraged to participate in the research programs of the centre.
5. The appointee will assist in teaching of undergraduates, postgraduates, MLSO and nursing staff, and participate in providing in service training programs for BTS staff.
6. The appointee will be required to provide cover for clinical and on-call duties during the absence of colleagues on leave etc.
7. The appointee will undertake other duties as required by the Regional Director.

Figure 1.

Entry to the consultant grade in the UK is controlled by limiting the number of designated training posts (career registrar/senior registrar) in each specialty. The required number is a matter of fierce debate, but is controlled by the Government; the standards are set by the profession. Firstly, each training post must have an approved training program with appropriate facilities available; this is approved by the Joint Committee of Higher Medical Education which has a Specialty Advisory Committee for each of the recognised disciplines with representatives from the Royal Colleges, national societies and distinguished consultants. Secondly, each candidate must obtain the appropriate specialty diploma (by examination) from the Royal Colleges of Physicians and/or Pathologists.

The criteria for entry to Transfusion Medicine are therefore now clearly (but not necessarily precisely) laid down, and the standards will be set and maintained by senior specialists in the field. However, exams are by themselves poor indicators of practical competence to practice as an independent consultant, and restructuring of the MRCPath. exam is taking place to allow more emphasis on practical aspects, including data interpretation and analysis, and less "book work". Nevertheless, the exam is perceived as a significant hurdle with written, laboratory practical and oral components, with a 50-60% pass rate at first attempt. A historical difficulty with Transfusion Medicine has been the lack of such an exam designed for the needs of those intending to practice exclusively in the specialty, with most trainees recruited from hematology, which only requires six months total exposure in blood transfusion, and the obligation to pass the entire hematology exam containing less than 10% relevant material.

In theory each trainee is supposed to have regular and frequent contact with the regional postgraduate committees responsible for supervision, to ensure adequate progress is being made and sufficient facilities are being made available. In practice these reviews are often less than satisfactory, with candidates not being advised about poor progress or prospects until very late, and much of the responsibility is left to the trainee's "chief" – who may himself be the problem!

More emphasis is now being placed on the quality of the training program and its content, and ensuring that the designated post is indeed used for training. The difficulty of ensuring an adequate balance between service, training and research is considerable due to increasing pressure of work, insufficient funding for meetings attendance etc. Nevertheless, considerable importance is attached to the "apprenticeship" system in the UK where the trainee learns by example, and by carrying out the full range of work/tasks under supervision in controlled safe circumstances – the consultant remains ultimately responsible for work carried out by junior staff. Ideally such posts should be "supernumerary" but must also be integrated into service and on-call work to ensure sufficient "hands-on" experience. In recognition of the need for continuous education, up to 30 days paid study leave may be granted over three years.

The above remains the ideal. Understaffing places pressures on both the trainee and supervisor; there are no formally designated trainers among consultants, and the task is approached with varying degrees of enthusiasm; accreditation is automatic provided the required amount of time has been spent in JCHMT approved posts; the training programs are rather vague with no clearly defined objectives; acceptability of training standards is limited to scrutiny of written submissions with episodic visits of JCHMT representatives to training establishments to assess facilities etc. Much is taken on trust rather than by formal procedure; yet in a typically British way the system works remarkably well and competition is generally fierce among the trainees, particularly in the popular specialties, and the standard attained (academically) is high.

Unfortunately there is a danger with rigidly defined specialty training programs in that those unable to attain a consultant post in their chosen specialty have few alternatives, since completion of accreditation and obtaining the required diploma does not in any way guarantee a consultant post, and more effort is required in selecting and monitoring trainees at the outset. Transfusion Medicine used to be the refuge of a number of hematology "drop-outs" because there was no separate training program and it seemed an easy option. Now that there is a separate JCHMT approved training program, and the Royal College of Pathologists is to set the MRCPath. (transfusion medicine) diploma exam, the only problem that remains is to attract sufficient high-calibre individuals to the training posts. Within the Scottish National Blood Transfusion Service, the opportunity has been taken to completely reorganize training programs in order to avoid the above problems; a key element is the rotation of senior registrars to another regional centre for approximately one year, and supervision of progress and performance by a training committee with representatives from each region.

It has to be said that the trainee specialists probably succeed in spite of the system, which tends to equate success with academic achievements, research papers, higher degrees (MD/PhD), and the passing of examinations, and the sound well-trained individual with considerable practical experience who is content to provide a good service is at a disadvantage in applying for consultant posts.

Training for, and entry to a specialty is relatively well defined in a number of European Economic Community (EEC) countries but nevertheless there remain a number of potentially contentious issues – who defines a "new" specialty such as Transfusion Medicine; what are the boundaries; how is overlap with existing specialties resolved; what about interprofessional rivalry and entrenched interests etc.? These must be resolved if acceptable training programs are to be defined and a relevant body of knowledge is to be acquired by the prospective specialist.

Accredited specialists (consultants)

In contrast to the closely regulated and controlled system for the training of specialists in the UK, career development and education for consultants is somewhat rudimentary and informal in the sense that there are no nationally prescribed training programs or update courses which are mandatory, and proof of attendance or the need to spend a given number of hours on continuing education is not a requirement to remain on the specialist register – indeed there are no specialist registers as such in the UK, although this is in the process of change with the GMC developing a voluntary system recording completion of specialist training. The newly appointed specialist is probably at the peak of all round theoretical and practical knowledge, but perhaps lacking in experience, particularly in organisation and management; thereafter progress is variable and idiosyncratic, depending on opportunity, resources and personal motivation. Depending on the appointment there will be a variable requirement for service routine, teaching, research administration etc. and in theory the job description should define these. In practice, until recently job descriptions were written with vague generalisations and rarely, if ever, revised and updated. This meant that consultants could, and did, create their own job resulting in "job drift" in response to clinical demands, or personal interest.

The situation in UK regional transfusion centres was probably better than most in that the regional director had overall responsibility for medical matters, with some authority (usually managerial) over colleagues – but this was very much the exception in hospital practice where all consultants are "equal" with clinical freedom to pursue their own cherished ideas and to develop their practice with very little interference. This approach is both a strength and a weakness in that stultifying uniformity is avoided, the energetic and enthusiastic could develop and introduce new techniques without "interference", and centres of excellence could develop; but on the other hand there were opportunities to avoid change, to indulge in non-productive activities, and so on, so that considerable variation in practices, unequal workloads, and other unplanned developments could take place. Government suspicion (largely unfounded) that many consultants were working less than contracted hours, wide variation in indicators such as waiting lists, length of hospital stay after various procedures, etc. led to the introduction of new consultant job descriptions and job plans in the new recently introduced NHS regulations.

Job descriptions and job plans

There can be little argument that reasonably clearly defined job descriptions are advantageous to both employer and employee. The difficulty arises in defining the content in such a way that it does not conflict with clinical responsibility for the patient, and reflects the realities of the degree of uncertainty in being in any one place at any one time. The new job plans (Figure 2) are quite detailed, including a weekly timetable of fixed commitments, and a break-

[   ] Health board
Recommended outline work program for consultant staff

Name:
Specialty:
Contract:*   Whole-time
                Maximum part-time
                Part-time ... NHDs
                Honorary ... NHDs
                (* delete as appropriate)

a. Weekly timetable of fixed commitments (i.e. regular scheduled NHS activities in accordance with paragraph 30b of the terms and conditions of service)

		Hospital/Other location	**Type of work**
Monday	am		
	pm		
Tuesday	am		
	pm		
Wednesday	am		
	pm		
Thursday	am		
	pm		
Friday	am		
	pm		
Weekend			

Note: Only fixed commitments should be included in this timetable.

b. Average number of hours spent each week on NHS duties

Type of duty	**Average number of hours**
Out-patients	
Ward work	
Theatre or special procedures	
Training/Teaching/Examining/Accredition	
Research	
Laboratory/Imaging services	
Medical Audit	
Management	
Committees (local or national)	
Administration	
Other duties (please specify)	
Travelling time (part-time only)	
On-call for emergency	
(Give rota arrangements – e.g. 1:4 and number of sites covered)	

Figure 2.

down of the average number of hours spent each week on a range of NHS duties including teaching, administration, research, on-call, etc. The significant departure from before is the need to specify in some detail the relative proportion of each type of activity, rather than vague generalities. This does pose some practical difficulties in a mainly laboratory based specialty such as Transfusion Medicine since there is no equivalent to an operating session or a ward round, and flexibility is required. The other new feature is the need to have the job plan agreed and countersigned by the general manager of the unit, and to be reviewed and updated on an annual basis. As yet we have no practical experience of this new system and there are understandable concerns that this could lead to undue pressure and restriction of professional freedom from heavy-handed managers; the best defence against this would be to do a good job and earn the respect of the managers. Only time will tell whether this system has the negative effect of actually minimising change and innovation and reduces individual incentive to improve and advance rather than just doing a basic job. Certainly, the completion of job plans has made most consultants realise that they are actually putting in far more hours of work than recognised, particularly in administration, paperwork and keeping up with the literature, which all too often gets done at home and at the week-ends.

Whereas the job plan gives a framework for *what* a consultant is supposed to do, it does not (yet?) specify *how* this should be done since this comes within professional responsibility.

Performance appraisal

The question of whether doctors are performing to an acceptable standard is a valid one to ask, but the means of defining the answer is one of the most contentious of medical topics. This is because there is no simple answer – each patient transaction is unique; local circumstances and resources must be taken into account; there may be genuine uncertainty and controversy about the "best" treatment, etc. – but we all think we can recognise "bad" practice. The difficulty is in agreeing objective standards which are applicable to all circumstances. A further difficulty is the jealously guarded concept of clinical freedom, associated with personal responsibility for the patient, which tends to make any adverse criticism of treatment "taboo", – ill-advised comment can be considered unprofessional conduct and may be an occasion for review by the GMC.

In a completely free market, the patients would ultimately decide whether a doctor's performance was acceptable and control standards by consulting only those giving a good service, and suing those who gave an unacceptable service, and only the "good" doctors would remain in business. This approach is not in the best interest of the patients since it is reactive rather than proactive, and it is better to avoid poor results than to correct them afterwards. It can also lead to patients "shopping around" to find a doctor unscrupulous enough to agree to the patients demands.

In business and management, appraisal of performance (AP) schemes have been in use for many years, particularly in large successful organisations. Their application has been largely restricted to managerial performance, with set targets and objectives designed for the marketplace, linked to financial rewards. The NHS reorganisation to introduce general management structures in the delivery of health care has also resulted in the introduction of AP for the new general managers, complete with salary incentives, in an effort to make the NHS more efficient and cost-effective. These schemes are now being applied to other health professionals, but the key question is whether they are applicable outside the strictly managerial framework where there is not only a clearly defined hierarchy of "bosses", but also a defined hierarchy of responsibilities as well – these are alien concepts to the practice of medicine at the consultant level.

The objectives of AP are laudable – to plan work, to set required measures of performance, to assess progress, and to actively develop managers and practitioners to their full potential in a continuous iterative process – the AP cycle (Figure 3). The central element is the appraisal interview between manager and subordinate, and there is no doubt that the AP framework could work well in a number of areas within the transfusion services – for example the achievement of blood collection targets, plasma targets, reporting of laboratory results within a certain time – but less satisfactorily where professional judgement is required. Potential conflict of interest and confrontation between manager and consultant is almost inevitable unless only the most broad of objectives is discussed. It is possible that the annual review of job plans for consultants will in fact evolve to a form of job appraisal, but only in general terms such as waiting lists, numbers of outpatients seen, laboratory specimens processed etc., perhaps with comparison of workload indicators between consult-

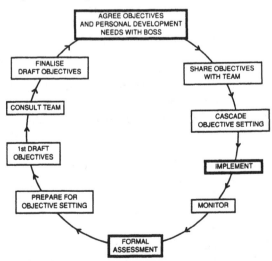

Figure 3. The AP cycle.

ants in the same specialty. But the dangers of comparing simple numbers, without considering complexity or outcome, are obvious to the medical profession, and it is doubtful whether non-medical managers are sufficiently qualified to make such judgements. In practice, it would appear that managers are delegating such tasks to clinical directors, heads of service, heads of department and similar senior medical staff, so that the success or otherwise initiatives rests with the medical profession.

The transfusion services in the UK are mainly organised through the regional centres, each with a regional director who is usually managerially as well as professionally responsible, and there is an opportunity to influence the introduction of review mechanisms so as to minimise conflict of interests; the most difficult aspect will be to agree standards against which performance should be measured.

Medical audit

Whereas the introduction of management techniques into consultant practice can improve organisational efficiency and communications and can reduce unnecessary waste, they do not resolve the most important issue of the appropriateness and outcome of the doctor-patient (or doctor-donor) interaction. Assessment and analysis of medical practice has formed the experimental test for the introduction of new practices, and the basis of medical education; the standards set by experts have always been a yardstick against which others could measure their own performance. Whereas the conscientious have always made the effort to keep up-to-date by attending lectures, clinical meetings, symposia etc. and by reading the appropriate specialist journals, there is no compulsion to do so. In any case, there is an inbuilt bias in the presentation of new medical information towards the academic and scientific acquisition of knowledge without equal regard for patient outcome, cost-effectiveness and similar issues – the application of "high-tech" medicine may be satisfying for the practitioners, but not necessarily more beneficial to the patient. Professional discussion of the investigation and management of "interesting cases" takes place at clinical meetings, grand rounds etc. but these cases are usually of academic interest rather than representative, and direct criticism of the quality of care or outcome is rare.

The new procedures introduced into the NHS by the government now include a formal mechanism of medical audit which has the objectives of "the systematic, critical analysis of the quality of medical care, including the procedures used for diagnosis, treatment, the use of resources, and the resulting outcome and quality of life for the patient". The formation of medical audit committees in the various specialties is now obligatory, although in fact many longstanding professional activities involving audit have been in place for years – e.g. the National Quality Control Scheme for Pathology Laboratories (begun in 1969) includes blood group serology and compatibility testing and makes each participating laboratory aware of its performance compared with

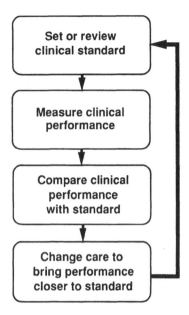

Figure 4. Medical audit cycle.

every other laboratory; many institutions have a hospital transfusion committee which reviews practices and makes recommendations. Apart from improving the quality and efficiency of patient care, medical audit is also a significant opportunity to enhance medical education by promoting discussion between colleagues about practice. To be beneficial, audit should lead to improvement; this is best achieved by systematic analysis – the "audit cycle" (Figure 2).

The setting of explicit standards is not easy but can enhance continuing medical education by focusing debate on the definition of specific goals and the means of achieving them. The confidential setting of medical audit, where both patient and doctor identity remains confidential, should encourage open peer review where there are deviations from the agreed standard, and the identification of bad practices (in terms of patient outcome). The new framework also allows the identification of the "persistent poor performer", with the offer of remedial action in the form of educational opportunities, or possibly additional resources.

However, it must be emphasised that the primary objective of medical audit is educational – to raise the performance of the average to the excellent. It is not intended as a tool for management to detect bad practice among medical staff, nor for disciplinary purposes; existing procedures are already established for dealing with the dangerous or sick doctor. The medical profession does recognise the need for some mechanism to review and deal with doctors who are neither of the above, but whose long-term fitness to practice is questionable. This most important issue is under active discussion by the GMC and

Royal Colleges, and also extends to the wider issues on the principles of definition of specialties, and of harmonisation within the EEC.

References

1. Appraisal and appraisal interviewing. The Industrial Society, London, 1985.
2. Appraisal of performance – Guide and Documentation, Management Development Group, Scottish Health Service, March 1990.
3. Hospital Medical and Dental Staff. Consultant's contracts and job plans. NHS Circular No. 1990(PCS)23.
4. Medical audit. Report of the Royal College of Physicians of London, March 1989.
5. Guidance on medical audit. NHS Circular No. 1989(GEN)29.

TRANSFUSION MEDICINE, EDUCATION AND THE COMMUNITY: DONOR MOTIVATION AND COMMUNITY ORIENTED ASPECTS

A.P.M. Los, C.Th. Smit Sibinga

Introduction

The basic consideration of this symposium is "fact and fiction in Transfusion Medicine". This basic consideration has been given a special meaning by the words Graham Greene wrote in his novel "Monsignor Quixote": "Facts and fictions: they are not always easy to distinguish" [1]. When there exists common agreement on the "truth" of a statement this will not automatically include whether it is a fact or a fiction. Man can agree or disagree both on the perceived truth of statements and define them as facts or as fictions. What is a fact for the one does not automatically mean a fact to the other, it might as well be a fiction. It would take another symposium to grasp the full philosophical meaning of the notions mentioned. Still it will be the question whether the full range of the concepts and their interaction will be completely understood.

Let us have a look at the value of the following statements in terms of facts or fictions: "The fundament of blood transfusion is the willingness of the community to share the blood", and "The willingness or motivation should be based on the concept of blood being a national resource to be shared by all". Even the two statements shown could be fictitious for some persons, however, in the rather limited world of blood bankers we would like to presume the truth of the statements to be accepted as a fact in any case.

However, the question is whether the consequences of the approval of these statements are generally understood. The consequence of common agreement on the truth of the statements shown, is a need for a special educational approach and mechanisms of continuous appeal of all groups in the society in order to achieve general acceptance in the society. All these efforts that have the ultimate goal to care for and to safeguard continuity, self-sufficiency and sustainability of the donor base can be reduced to the common denominator: "donor management". Thus, specific educational research and mechanisms to reach the community are important aspects of "donor management".

We feel that it is a fiction to believe that such a comprehensive and fundamental approach on donor management is generally accepted and applied.

It can not be denied that donor management is largely situated in a primarily good willing but rather amateuristic corner. It is not our intention to question the integrity and dedication of blood bank employees involved in the field of donor recruitment and/or donor management. The term amateuristic should therefore not be regarded as unfavourable, but rather as a synonym of unsystematic, unscientific, and insufficient evaluation. Of course there has been done an abundance of research on aspects of blood donation and donor management, however no doubt there has been a one-sided attention on the motivation of becoming a blood donor. In the literature on blood donation we find the majority of articles on this specific subject. The American scientist R.M. Oswalt, who did much research on donor motivation, even wonders whether it is still necessary to do research on the motivation of donors and non-donors, since it is questionable whether there has been some change in these fundamental characteristics of men, especially of those who give their blood for fellow human beings. Oswalt suggests that "additional surveys of blood donor and non-donor motivations are not likely to produce any significant new information since essentially the same information has been forthcoming for the last twenty years or so" [2].

Thus, the fundament of donor management should be more extensive, and not only involve research on motivation of donors per se.

The most important and continuous thread in donor management should be the establishment and maintenance of a relationship between donor and blood bank, which may result in awareness of personal responsibility, since this is starting point for a safe and reliable blood supply.

In donor management a number of important aspects should be distinguished, which should get equal attention: characteristics of first-time donors, donor selection, the period donors are "active" (length of the "donor career"), the characteristics of resigned donors, the reasons for resignation and deferral, and the way donors perceive the given information.

When "Transfusion Medicine" as a discipline is regarded as an aim to bring together, canalize and aggregate the available "know how" on the therapeutic application of blood and blood components, then a professional and scientific approach of donor management should have an important place. Donor management is too important to be approached on an unprofessional, unsystematic, and unscientific way. Donor management should be based on good scientific documentation, monitoring, and evaluation. Fundamental in this approach is a good notion and insight in the characteristics and composition of the population from which the donors could be recruited and selected, and the characteristics and composition of the existing donor population. It is a fact that these characteristics differ from place to place and from country to country. Second, good knowledge of the way persons (donors and non-donors) perceive the given information is needed, since the comprehension of the information provided and the messages given is of paramount importance. Both aspects mentioned are of equal importance and are complementary, because before we can reach the community we should have sufficient insight in the characteristics of the community. The "message" should fit each target group in a taylor-made fashion and should be given by adequate information materials.

The scientific basis for this approach should therefore be twofold: First there should be research on the characteristics of the community, and second there should be research on the ways how to reach the community.

Characteristics of the community

The first community oriented aspect to be worked out is the need for basic demographic information of the communities of interest: The general population and the donor population. Important questions to be asked are: What data do we need, what is the availability of data, and how should the data be collected and registered.

General population

Fundamental basic information is needed on demographic characteristics of the general population from which the donor population should be recruited.

In the western world we presume there are population registers on different levels (country, province, city, etc.). From these registers the basic information on population demographics could be available. However, it should be realised that this basic information is not available worldwide. Registration by census has yet to be implemented in many countries. For a basic demographic description of the general population the following data could be sufficient: Number, gender, age, domicile. However, the availability of additional data could provide more possibilities for gaining insight and knowledge of the general population, the source of future donors.

As an example, the results of studies on the characteristics of the general population and donor population in the region of the Red Cross Blood Bank Groningen-Drenthe, NL (RCBBG-D) will be presented [3].

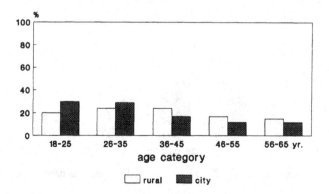

Figure 1. Age distribution general population; rural population Groningen-Drenthe and city of Groningen (NL).

100

In the Netherlands there does exist opportunity for access to the demographics of the general population. From the Dutch population registers unique data are available to describe the general population by age, city size, and gender [4].

The total population in the area (region Groningen-Drenthe and the city of Groningen) comprises over 680,000 persons in the age of 18-65 years. Figure 1 shows the age distribution of the general population in the rural area of the region Groningen-Drenthe (over 562,000 population in the age of 18-65 years), and the city of Groningen (over 118,000 population in the age of 18-65 years). The male-female ratio in the general population is about 1:1. The distribution of the city population has a bias towards the younger age categories, compared with the rural population.

Donor population

Starting point for the availability of donor data is an optimal and continuous registration of demographic characteristics of the donor population. This need for basic demographic information comprises not only the characteristics of the actual active donor base, but also characteristics of first-time donors, donors who resign, i.e. the deferred donors, from which the reason for deferring is known, donors who quit for unknown reasons, and the length of the donor career.

The donor population of the RCBBG-D is registered in a computer data base. From the latter data base the variables gender, postal code and age were selected from each donor. From postal code the domicile (rural or urban) of the donor was determined.

In the donor base over 50,000 donors are registered: Over 40,000 in the rural area, and over 10,000 in the city of Groningen.

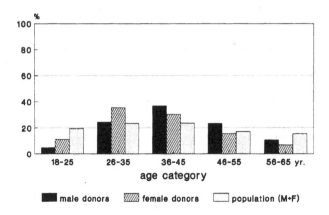

Figure 2. Donor and non-donor population; by age and gender (rural area).

In the following figures some basic demographic characteristics of the donor population in the region of the RCBBG-D are presented. For a good overview the relevant characteristics of the general population, which were presented in Figure 1, are included.

Figure 2 shows the age distribution of the rural donor population by gender. The male-female ratio in the rural donor population is about 1.3:1. The size of the different age groups of rural donors differs from the general rural population. The youngest age group (18-25 years) and the oldest age group (56-65 years) show a relative underrepresentation of donors. In addition there is a difference in age distribution of male and female donors.

Figure 3 shows the age distribution of the donor population in the city of Groningen. The age distribution of the urban donor population differs from the age distribution of the rural donor population. Like the shift to the younger age categories in the general population, there is a shift to the younger age categories, both for the male and female donors. The male-female ratio in the donor population of the city of Groningen is about 1.1:1.

When the demographic characteristics of the donor population are compared with the characteristics of the general population we would conclude that both in the rural area and in the city of Groningen, for both sexes, there is a relative underrepresentation of the younger age group. Furthermore, there does exist a difference in composition between male and female donor population. In general the female donor population is younger than the male donor population. This brings us to the question of the origin of these results. Three factors determine the development of the composition of the donor population: 1) the composition of the first-time donor population; 2) the demographic composition of the resigned and deferred donor population; 3) the length of the donor career.

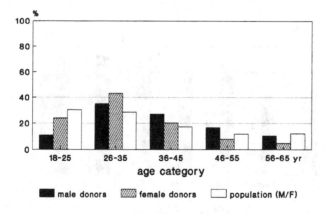

Figure 3. Donor and non-donor population; by age and gender (city).

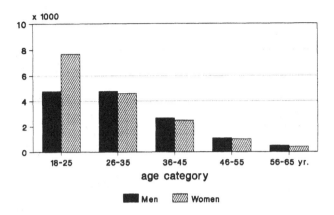

Figure 4. First-time donors 1983-1989; by gender and age.

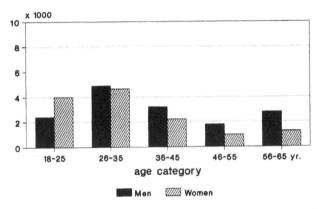

Figure 5. Resignations and deferrals 1983-1989; by gender and age.

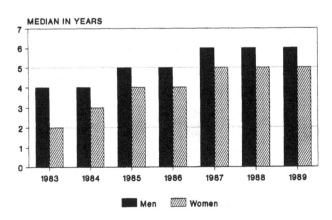

Figure 6. Donor career 1983-1989; by gender.

First-time donors

Figure 4 shows the age distribution of first-time donors by gender (in the period 1983-1989). There is a striking difference in the composition by gender of first-time donors. It is not surprising that the first-time donor population is relatively young. However, in the youngest age category there are almost twice as many female than male donors.

Resigned and deferred donors

Figure 5 gives an overview of the resignations and deferrals in the same period. The difference between male and female first-time donors in the youngest age category seems to be compensated by the difference in the resignation in the youngest category. There are more females than males resigning. We would conclude that there are relatively more first-time female donors than first-time male donors in the youngest age group. However, the "loss" by resignation and deferral of female donors in this age group is also higher than the "loss" of male donors.

Donor career

Figure 6 illustrates that female donors show a shorter donor career than male donors, although an increase is noticed for both sexes over the period 1983-1989. This results is in concurrence with the presented differences between male and female donors.

From the presented results we can conclude that there is a difference in the donor profile of male and female donors. In general the female first-time donor is younger, but has a shorter donor career than the male donor. So, from these basic demographic characteristics we can conclude that specific attention should be given to the length of the donor career, and the difference in donor career between men and women. Insight in these matters could be beneficial for retention of donors. More extensive study on these characteristics over a certain time-period, in other words time analysis of the development of the demographic composition of the general population and the donor population (first-time, active, resigned) could signalize relevant trends and form a basis for donor policy.

Reasons for resignation and deferral

No doubt, the basic demographic characteristics (basic data) of blood donors should be supplemented with data on the specific reasons for becoming a blood donor (motivation to become a blood donor). However, special attention and emphasis should be given to the specific reasons for remaining a blood donor (motivation to continue donating blood), and the specific reasons for deferring and/or quitting the donor base i.e. the reasons for resigning. A recent study at the RCBBG-D on the reasons for resignation and deferral showed a deficiency in our knowledge on this specific subject as is shown in the next figures.

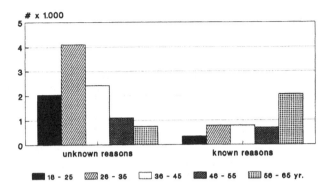

Figure 7. Resignations and deferrals 1983-1989; known/unknown reasons by age. Male donors

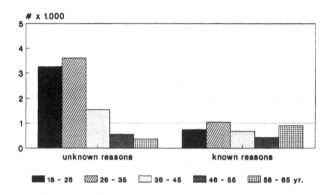

Figure 8. Resignations and deferrals 1983-1989; known/unknown reasons by age. Female donors

Figure 7 shows that the majority of resignations is for unknown reasons and for male donors a prevalence in the age group 26-35 years.

Figure 8 shows that also for female donors the majority of resignations is for unknown reasons and even more distinct in the youngest age groups.

These results suggest again a special attention to be focused on the youngest age groups. In this case special attention on the specific reasons for resignation and the length of donor career, in other words on retention of (female) donors.

Reaching the community

Let us focus now on the second aspect of the proposed scientific approach on donor management. The crucial question here is how to reach the community.

A fundamental theoretical basis for this approach could be found in early American sociology, especially in the thoughts of the sociologist William I. Thomas (1863-1947). Thomas is the fourth and last of the early American sociologists whose works remain as relevant and important today as when they were written. Above anyone else Thomas gave fertile emphasis to the fact that in human behaviour it is not the objective situation that leads to social action but the individuals' perception and definition of the situation. His famous theorem reads: "If men define situations as real, they are real in their consequences" [4].

The truth and the impact of this theorem was illustrated when the Last National Bank (USA, 1932) was confronted with a rumour that there was shortage of money. The clients defined the situation as real, went "en masse" to the bank and asked for their money. Of course there was not enough stock to satisfy everybody and the bank broke: this was the consequence of defining a fictitious situation as real, also defined as "self-fulfilling prophecy" [6]. Applying this natural law on the theme of this symposium it could be said that a fiction results in a fact; for the bank an undesired fact.

The individuals' perception and definition of the situation leads to social action. Applying Thomas' theorem on donor management it should be clear that an important goal of donor management should be to achieve general agreement and acceptance of the statements mentioned: "The fundament of blood transfusion is the willingness of the community to share the blood", and "The willingness or motivation should be based on the concept of blood being a national resource to be shared by all". It should also be clear that donor management based on good scientific documentation and evaluation can prevent rumours to get a chance and that we will be confronted with uncontrolled and undesired facts.

Thoroughly designed, monitored and evaluated programs on donor management should result in a common believe, and acceptance in the society of the two statements mentioned, and hence, according to the natural law formulated by Thomas, result in a real consequence and desired fact: A sufficient, reliable, and sustainable blood supply for the future. However, necessary condition is profound research on the efficacy of the instruments of communication that play an important role in the fundamental aspects of donor management: Motivation and selection of first-time donors (reaching the general population), motivation and selection of "active" donors, and prevention of unnecessary resignations (reaching the donor population).

General population

Starting point is motivation and selection of first-time donors, and thus reaching the general population. The instrument to reach the community is the "message" that should suit each target group in a taylor-made fashion and should be given by adequate information materials. Research on the characteristics of the community should provide us with sufficient information on the demographic composition of the different target groups. A relative under-representation of for instance certain age groups can be signalized through comparison of donor population and general population. Thus, special attention can be given to these categories of potential donors. No doubt the more information available of the population, the better the message can be adjusted to the categories of interest. For example additional information on the level of education, and professional status of the population could be helpful to make the message suit properly. Some important aspects of donor motivation and donor recruitment could be summarized as follows: First there should be emphasis on personal responsibility to support and contribute. Blood donation should be voluntary but not without engagement. Second, adequate information and enlightment should be given, and most important final point: The language used should be simple, clear and metaphorical. A repeat use of short slogans has proven its efficacy in many advertisement campaigns!

In the past tremendous efforts have been undertaken to recruit first-time donors. The abundance of presentations on this field during the Third International Colloquium on the Recruitment of Voluntary Blood Donors (Hannover, August 1990) showed a great variety of measures taken to recruit and motivate persons to become blood donor [6]. The measures varied from well designed educational programs for young people at schools to the use of mass media, such as regular publications in the news papers that show the actual situation of the blood supply (stock) and the actual need (shortage) if present. However, despite this abundance of proposed measures and measures effectuated, often the sigh was heard: "We do not now what the real effect of our program is on the long run". This is exactly what seems to happen over and over again. The programs sound very good, the results can be seen on short term, however there is little or no insight in the effects (efficacy) of the measures on the long run. It seems relatively easy to win first-time donors, especially with hard-marketing techniques. However, the problem is how to retain them and guarantee continuity of blood donation. There is little long-term planning and an absence of adequate monitoring and evaluation of the measures taken.

It is a fact: There is often direct visibility of donor recruitment programs. However, the efficacy of these taken measures on the long run could be fictitious. There is a need for more insight in "long term" effects and efficacy of given information materials and/or information methods used in reaching the community and target groups. In other words a need for adequate scientific monitoring and evaluation of measures taken to reach the general population.

Donor population

This need for adequate scientific monitoring and evaluation does not decline when recruitment and motivation has been successful and persons have become blood donor. There should also be research on the efficacy of the instrument of communication that plays a role in the continuation of motivation and selection of first-time donors, the continuation of motivation and selection of "active" donors, and the retention of "active" donors, in other words the prevention of unnecessary resignation.

Motivation and selection of first-time donors

First-time donors should get adequate information of all relevant aspects of donorship. The most important and continuous thread should be the establishment of a relationship between donor and blood bank, which should result in awareness of personal responsibility, as the fundament for a safe and reliable blood supply.

Recruitment of potential donors does not seem to be the major problem. However, the bottle neck is the selection and retention of first-time donors and regular donors.

Motivation and selection of "active" donors

There are many options to provide adequate information. However, we have our doubts on the efficacy of written information materials. In the near past two surveys were carried out in the RCBBG-D (1985, 1987) to evaluate the impact of given information materials on AIDS and risk factors [8]. The most important results showed that, although a majority confirms receiving the information materials on AIDS and risk factors (a personally addressed letter was used), there seem to be little comprehension on the specific subject. Furthermore there seemed to be an increase of irritation being confronted with apparently similar information each time again when coming to the blood bank to donate blood. Most donors did not feel the information was applicable to them.

More dramatically, as confirmed in the literature, it is a fact that regular donors keep on giving blood while carrying a risk factor for HIV transmission despite all available and provided information on the subject. So, it is a fiction to believe that the available written information is adequate and properly read. It is also a fiction to believe that there exists a general awareness of personal responsibility. Recently, the RCBBG-D was confronted with three HIV seroconversions. All three related to regular donors who apparently denied or suppressed the given information on risk factors.

This brings us again to the need of scientific research on the mechanisms that play a role, the need for implementation of this knowledge in policies, and a need for proper monitoring and evaluation of the measures taken.

Prevention on unnecessary resignation

Information on demographic characteristics and reasons for deferral over the period 1983-1989 (Figures 7 and 8) showed the majority of resignation being for unknown reasons, particularly in the youngest age categories, especially young female donors. At this moment we have no insight in the real motives of those who quit the donor base for unknown reasons. Further research is needed on this subject. It suggests that an important aspect of donor management should be attention on the retention of donors, and prevention of unnecessary resignation.

Aspects of educational process

Fundamental aspects of an educational process are published in the Educational Handbook for Health Personnel, published by the WHO [9]. These aspects could form a guideline for a general approach of donor management. The aspects are: Objective, assessment of need, planning, implementation, monitoring and evaluation.

Two main objectives and assessments of need are formulated: First the need for insight and knowledge of mechanisms of donor selection, mechanisms that prevent donors from refraining from donation when necessary, and second mechanisms how to prevent donors from unnecessary resignation: How to retain regular donors.

The third item suggests proper planning of measures. At the RCBBG-D the implementation of structured "exit interviews" or "exit questionnaires" is considered to gain more insight in the resignations for unknown reasons. On the basis of this specific information, programs should be designed with emphasis on retainment of regular donors. The effect and efficacy of the taken measures can be monitored through systematic and periodical research on the development of the demographic composition of the donor population, and especially the change in number of characteristics of the resigned and deferred donors. The results from these regular follow-up studies on donor demographics should be evaluated and lead to adjustment of the taken measures.

Final remark

It will be clear that all proposed aspects of donor management can not properly be implemented without personal commitment, efforts and funds. In the Netherlands we are still depending on the modest possibilities of blood bank budgets and on incidental grants from the government, which time after time has to be persuaded and impressed of the necessity of fundamental research on all aspects of donor management mentioned.

All aspects of donor management need adequate implementation in a national or even international infrastructure. When donor management is taken as a serious part of Transfusion Medicine there should also be funds to give structure to the organisation (national and international) of the research facilities. We therefore strongly agree with professor Jane Piliavin who, at the end of her excellent overview of the research on blood donors since 1977, suggests a timely development of a new research foundation to support both basic and applied research, funded by all of the major organisations in the field [10].

Conclusions

There is a need for structural funds to create the conditions under which the research on scientific documentation, monitoring and evaluation can be implemented.

World wide, country by country, registration of the general and donor population should be implemented and is a necessary condition for further research on donor management.

For full profit of demographics of general and donor population there is need for additional data on the educational level of the community, and their profession and/or professional status.

The emphasis in donor management should be on selection and retention. There is need for specific research on reasons for resignation and deferral, and thus mechanisms of retention of donors.

Keywords are the establishment and maintenance of a relationship between donor and blood bank, and the achievement of personal responsibility.

All measures taken in the field of donor management should be subject to scientific monitoring and evaluation.

References

1.Green G. Monsignor Quixote. Pinguin Books 1984.
2.Oswalt RM. A review of blood donor motivation and recruitment. Transfusion 1977;17:123-35.
3.Central Bureau of Statistics. Voorburg, The Netherlands.
4.Los APM, Lumey LH. Risicofactoren voor (overdracht van) HIV-infectie: Verschillen tussen bloeddonoren en niet-donoren. Deel I: Demografie donoren en algemene bevolking. RIVM, Bilthoven 1990.
5.Thomas WI, Thomas DS. The child in America. Alfred Knopf, New York 1928.
6.Merton RK. Social theory and social structure. The Free Press, New York 1986.
7.Proceedings of the IIIrd International Colloquium on the Recruitment of Voluntary Blood Donors, Hannover 1990. League of Red Cross and Red Crescent Societies, Geneva 1991.
8.Los APM, Achterhof L, Tijmstra Tj, Suurmeyer ThPBM, Smit Sibinga CTh. Informing blood donors about AIDS and risk factors: Reactions to information provided in a regional blood bank in the Neterlands. Aids 1989;3:439-41.
9.Educational Handbook for Health Personnel. WHO, Geneva 1987.
10.Piliavin JA. Why do they give the gift of life? A review of the research on blood donors since 1977. Transfusion 1990;30:444-59.

RESEARCH AND DEVELOPMENT PROGRAMS

J.E. Menitove

Introduction

The mission statement of most regional blood centers indicates their commitment to service and education; some also pursue research and/or development programs. A decision to concentrate on one or a combination of these aspects resides with a center's senior management and the board of directors. Obviously, all blood centers provide service: collection, processing and distribution of blood and components, often in conjunction with therapeutic apheresis services, red cell reference laboratories and rare donor registries. Some centers enhance their service commitment by including educational functions: Teaching and training, etc. for professionals and the public.

A minority of centers consider research and development programs integral to their missions. The commitment of top management is needed to insure the full support and nurturing that is required for a successful research program. Product development initiatives require a similar degree of guidance and attention. This essay includes: A definition of research and development; a description of highly successful industrial research and development programs; a discussion of research and development programs at blood centers; a list of factors and contribute to the success of research and development programs; and an explanation of potential benefits and risks these programs pose to blood centers.

Research

The dictionary defines research as careful, systematic study and investigation in some field of knowledge. It is assumed this includes basic and applied investigation. Basic science researchers seek fundamental discovery. They also teach and train new investigators. Applied research scientists pursue basic research but focus on producing new products and technology [1].

Why should a blood center have a research program? To Leon W. Hoyer, M.D., National Research Director, American Red Cross Blood Services, "Research and development programs are an integral part of American Red

Cross Blood Services. In sponsoring these programs, the Red Cross seeks to ensure donor safety, produce safer and more effective products for patients, and reduce costs through greater efficiency" [2]. Robert R. Montgomery, M.D., Director of Research, Blood Center of Southeastern Wisconsin, is convinced, "To not do research is to be satisfied with the status quo" [3].

Development involves the translation of research results into products, processes and services [4]. The focus is on product development and technology commercialization. Ian M. Ross, Ph.D., President of American Telephone and Telegraph Bell Laboratories, considers technology "the totality of means employed to provide objects necessary for human sustenance and comfort" [5]. For AT&T, the "need to communicate yields information technology".

Examples of corporate research and development programs

Research programs at two corporate leaders exemplify strategies taken by successful enterprises. Bell Laboratories is the paradigm of an industrial research center that relies on inhouse research for new products and technologies. Monsanto, Inc. a multinational corporation, on the other hand, formed a unique partnership with Washington University of St. Louis in the early 1980s to diversify into biotechnology-based products. While these approaches are quite disparate, they demonstrate the planning and vision taken by management to remain at the forefront, ahead of the competition.

Bell Laboratories

The American Telephone and Telegraph (AT&T) mission is to fulfil the need for human beings to communicate with each other. Since the initial experiments performed by Alexander Graham Bell and Thomas A. Watson in the early 1870s, the Bell System operated on the theory that research and development would yield improved communication. The motive for seeking improvements in technology combined scientific curiosity with corporative objectives. The Bell Companies wanted to retain their leading role in communications technology in the United States when Bell's original telephone patents ran out in the early 1990s. Under a series of legal agreements the fledgling Bell System Companies forged an agreement making Western Electric their sole supplier of equipment in 1882. By 1907 Western Electric integrated its manufacturing staff with AT&T's central engineering staff.

This action closed the gap between engineers working in the shops and those involved in pure science, thus aiding technology transfer [6]. The Bell System operated under the working principle that it would supply its own innovations without waiting for developments from the outside.

Also in 1907, Theodore H. Vail became the new head of AT&T. He was a pioneer in public relations, i.e. relations between the public and the corporation. He demanded honest reporting of the company's activities to the public. He also promoted the concept of "universality: One policy, one system, one universal service" [6]. He felt that competition between duplicate telephone systems within cities, which was prevalent at that time, was "wasteful" and led to duplication of central offices, charges, etc.

Vail wrote about the "served" and the "server". In the 1910 AT&T annual report he said: "There has always been and will always be the laudable desire of the great public to be served rightly and as cheaply as possible, which, sometimes selfishly degenerates into a lack of consideration for the rights of those who are served" [6]. He "contended that if there is to be no competition, there should be public control" [6]. As such, in 1910 Vail sought a permanent commission that would exercise control and regulation but would not manage, operate or dictate.

By 1925, laboratories that developed systems for amplifying telephone conversations, the high vacuum tube and the radio telephone, were reorganized into the Bell Laboratories, whose mission was to be the nidus for all knowledge and understanding needed for the advancement of communication facilities and systems. Interestingly, this was in strong contrast to the policies of the telephone company's new president, Walter S. Gifford. He felt the company should concentrate on telephone service and let other interests (such as radio) be managed by others. Gifford allowed Bell Laboratories to pursue research in the music industry with eventual production of talking pictures such as *Don Juan* in 1926 and *The Jazz Singer* in 1927. Subsequently, Bell Laboratories produced the transistor, the laser, the solar cell, advances in the science of radio astronomy, and is now involved in photonics (lightwave communications), microelectronics, hardware and software for speach synthesis and recognition, and networking and imaging [7-9].

Prior to divestiture, Bell Laboratories received support in the form of an assessment of approximately $.50 per telephone and revenues from Western Electric. After the breakup, funding has been derived from AT&T's corporate budget (basic research) and business revenues (development) [7].

Monsanto Company

During the 1980s Monsanto made a decision to significantly restructure its businesses by developing a presence in the biotechnology sector. It invested $150 million to construct a research facility in suburban St. Louis and hired a force of approximately 900 scientists. In 1982, it formed a unique partnership with Washington University of St. Louis in which Monsanto contributed $23.5 million over a 5-year period in exchange for leads in development of human pharmaceuticals [1].

Under the agreement, patents of all discoveries would be held by Washington University; however, Monsanto would have the first right to exclusive licenses under the patents. Individual researchers were not allowed to retain private rewards. All publications would be reviewed by Monsanto attorneys to determine whether they contained patentable discoveries; but the review process could not exceed 30 days. Hence, Monsanto's interest in obtaining product leads was protected without inhibiting those pursuing research interests.

It was felt that true collaboration between scientists at the two organizations would enhance technology transfer. For example, discovery of a protein with a specific physiological activity by a Washington University investigator might lead to collaboration with a Monsanto researcher with expertise in molecular biology. In turn, the protein would be cloned and expressed leading to further basic research.

On the downside, there was concern that the University's mission to conduct basic research would be a diverted to commercialization and would detract from its autonomy. In fact, Monsanto recognized the need for publications from academic departments and the turnaround time for the review process has been rapid. The agreement was renewed in 1986 and funding increased to approximately $62 million. It was subsequently extended through 1994 with a total investment of $100 million over the anticipated 12-year agreement.

Significant leads have been produced, 16 patents have been granted and 24 are pending, but as of 1991 there have been no products. Although disappointing, it may reflect the relatively long development period needed for pharmaceutical products rather than a failure of the initially proposed program goals.

Currently, Monsanto supports 50 research products that involve 120 Washington University scientists. There appears to be a long-range commitment and a belief that a mutually beneficial partnership has been forged. The two parties were able to agree on the purpose of the agreement, the benefits expected by both sides, the administrative structure, the details for financing the various phases, the procedure for review of publications and scientific findings, the patenting and licensing of scientific findings, issues of confidentiality, trade secrets and ownership, and procedures for amending the agreement. Overall they feel they have both "successfully capitalized on the strengths of each other to further the progress of science" [1].

Examples of blood center research and development programs; biomedical research and development: American Red Cross

The Jerome H. Holland Laboratory for Biomedical Sciences opened in February 1987 and serves as the headquarters laboratory of the American Red Cross Blood Services. Ten research laboratory and three service laboratory functions are housed in the Holland Laboratories. The research laboratories include biochemistry, immunology, cell biology, molecular biology, biology, plasma derivatives, product development, transplantation, transmissible diseases, and HLA. The service laboratories provide infectious disease testing, blood serology testing and reagent production [2].

The laboratories "demonstrate the Red Cross commitment ... to basic and applied research that is a critical part of (their) responsibility to blood donors and to the recipients of blood and blood components" [2]. An additional portion of the research and development program of the American Red Cross is conducted at the regional blood centers. Studies involving blood collection, testing, and distribution are more directly related to applied research efforts for improving services. Regional staff investigators work alongside clinicians prescribing blood and components. Several have close working relationships with hospitals and medical schools; collaborative efforts including basic research projects with these institutions have been encouraged. There is an investigator-initiated research project matching fund program available to assist regional staff to initiate new projects that have been approved by competitive review.

The Blood Center of Southeastern Wisconsin

Research has been an integral part of the Blood Center of Southeastern Wisconsin's programs since its inception in 1947. Currently the research staff is divided into four sections reflecting the interests of its senior investigators: Transfusion Medicine, hemostasis and platelet research and immunogenetics [10]. Over the years, basic research discoveries have been transferred into clinical laboratory tests and services. For example, the center's interest in HLA serology was extended into development of an extensive file of HLA-typed donors who readily consent to provide apheresis platelets for alloimmunized patients. More recently, these donors have been asked to be unrelated marrow donors for patients with life threatening illnesses for whom marrow transplantation is considered the only chance for survival. Research seeking an understanding of platelet immunology and pathogenesis of immune thrombocytopenic conditions led to establishment of a platelet antibody laboratory. Likewise, an interest in hemophilia and proteins involved in regulation of blood clotting led to establishment of a regional hemostasis laboratory. Tests are performed that are not available elsewhere in the community, such as von Willebrand multimer analysis and, protein C and protein S assays. Expertise in molecular biology led to the development of sequence specific oligonucleotide probe assays for HLA antigens and subsequent establishment of a service laboratory for molecular typings of HLA class II molecules for patients undergoing marrow transplantation.

Funding for research is derived from successful competition for National Institutes of Health, American Heart Association, etc. grants. A small portion is generated from the Center's Research Foundation; a for-profit subsidiary formed to generate income for research. The Center's Clinical Laboratories (including the Histocompatibility and Immunogenetics Laboratory, Paternity Testing Laboratory, Regional Hemostasis Labatory Platelet Antibody Labatory and DNA Typing Laboratories) currently account for almost 20% of the Center's annual budget. These laboratories are a diverse outgrowth of basic research investigations and represent successful technology transfer by a regional blood center.

New York Blood Center

The research arm of the New York Blood Center is the Lindsley F. Kimball Research Institute [11]. Its mission is to enhance the safety and efficacy of blood transfusion and to perform research about blood-related diseases. It has eighteen separate laboratories that study virology, blood coagulation biochemistry, biochemistry of red cell antigens, molecular analyses of blood group genes, epidemiology, membrane biochemistry and hematopoietic growth factors. Previously, work done at the institute was instrumental in identifying the hepatitis B agent and in conducting studies on the safety and efficacy of the hepatitis B vaccine.

Melville Biologics began as a research department and processes over 400,000 liters of plasma annually into albumin, gammaglobulin and factor-VIII concentrates. In conjunction with the Kimball Institute, it developed, patented and licensed the Blood Center's solvent detergent process for viral inactivation. In collaboration with pharmaceutical companies it is pursuing development and production of virus inactivated immunoglobulins, hemoglobin solutions as possible blood substitutes, fibronectin eye drops for corneal ulcers, platelet derived growth factor for wound-healing and development of an AT III concentrate.

Puget Sound Blood Center

The Puget Sound Blood Center Program in Seattle, Washington provides another example of a regional blood center with a research program. Since the early 1950s it has maintained close ties with the University of Washington, Division of Hematology. Under the auspices of the University, research was fostered and the academic careers of faculty were monitored. Significant contributions to blood banking and transfusion medicine have been made in the preparation and storage of red blood cells, platelet concentrates and cryoprecipitate. In addition, the knowledge about the genetics of blood groups and blood proteins has been expanded, treatment advance have occurred for patients with antiplatelet antibodies, the chemistry and biology of clotting factor proteins have been investigated and transplantation immunology studies have been undertaken. Transfusion safety research is conducted in patients with hemophilia who were infected with HIV or other viruses by blood components in the early 1980s. And, clinical research to determine if erythropoietin can be used to increase the volume of autologous blood prior to surgery was evaluated [12,13].

The center's clinical programs reflect the research interests of the senior investigators. From its onset in 1945, it provided a centralized crossmatching laboratory and clinical transfusion service to the hospitals it served. More than 400 patients with hemophilia in Washington, are under the auspices of a program that provides education and medical consultation to individuals, families, and physicians. The Center also maintains a coagulation laboratory, platelet antibody laboratory, outpatient transfusion clinic (including transfusion of hemophilia patients with cryoprecipitate) and an apheresis patient care service. The Center provides regional and national transplantation services, including an extensive listing of potential unrelated marrow donors and a histocompatibility laboratory that performs HLA typing, crossmatching and antibody screening for solid organ transplantation and bone marrow transplantation.

Contributing factors for successful research programs

Successful research programs do not occur by accident. Superior management skills of senior staff are essential. The ability to bring focus to a program and recruit innovative and creative scientists who work together to form a critical mass requires inordinate talent. Long-term planning, commitment, and resources (space, equipment and financing) are requisite. Productivity (publications) must be measured, acceptable performance judged by peer review (grants) must be defined and an appropriate compensation system must be established. To do this one must understand the motivation of scientists and their psychological traits.

Motivation of research scientists

Scientists are awed by challenge. Superior scientists are curious and creative and apply these talents to that challenge. They seek to put things in their place and derive significant satisfaction from knowing they are contributing to the state of knowledge. In general, they love competition and find peer recognition insatiable. They enjoy high incomes and the social status of being successful in their jobs [14].

Psychological traits of research scientists

In general, scientists are "thing" oriented. As a result they may relate poorly to other people. They are dedicated to a discipline as opposed to being "organization-conscious". Many scientists are resentful of authority, have one-track minds related to their competitive natures, display the "colleague syndrome" and for the most part are adverse to management roles.

The "colleague syndrome" reflects a scientist's tendency to disregard management as a discipline because it is not considered a true science. Investigators often do no respect superiors who lack scientific credentials. Affiliation with academic institutions is critical for many scientists. They are stimulated by peer interaction and, in the current high technology atmosphere, a critical mass of talent is required.

Scientists are often accused of being arrogant, selfish, myopic, uncommunicative, forgetful, and inconsiderate. They are concerned about people only when someone threatens their progress or when someone has the potential to facilitate their work.

Management of research scientists

Perhaps it is a myth to think that scientists can be managed; instead, their contributions can be maximized through encouragement, reward and tolerance. In fact "well-behaved" scientists who fit nicely into an organization are often bed scientists [15]. Hence, it is important to impose minimal boundaries and restrictions. Once they are instituted, they need to be made as clear as possible.

Noting the motivational factors of scientists, tangible and intangible rewards should be provided. This includes the fulfilment of money, space and equipment needs as well as appropriate support staff and involvement in a conducive milieu. Scientists should also be afforded maximum freedom in setting research priorities.

Integral to managing scientists is having superiors with the right credentials. If a scientist does not have respect for a supervisor, chaos is inevitable. A director of research sets the tone for an organization. He or she provides a "vision" and indirectly highlights the personal achievement of subordinate scientists. The director also receives credit if he is successful in guiding and imparting his knowledge to fledgling researchers. Peer recognition for the director and the research groups translates into an ability to attract new talent.

Creation of conducive milieu for research

Not only does a director of research have to understand how to manage a scientist, he must know how to create a milieu conducive to productive research. As already stated, the director must have the right credentials. Space, equipment, and money for program development and start-up or interim funding must be available. It is important to have proper academic affiliations. A conducive milieu has a critical mass of investigators who have interactive interests such that new discoveries are not isolated but instead provide the ground work for an explosion of excitement and creativity. Establishment of full-time positions with sufficient time to devote to research serves to minimize distractions. Without "protected time", scientists can feel over-burdened and may succumb to institutional rather than personal demands.

Contributory factors for successful development programs; motivation of developmental personnel

Those involved in development are more attuned to social needs of society. They are "need or achievement oriented". They are flexible and quick and adjust their approaches based on results. They enjoy tangible personal rewards, recognition, power, and independence, as well as money. Since they want to achieve technological contributions they may not quit when others with only financial goals would be deterred [15].

They understand that the innovative process is incremental and that new developments build on previous observations. As such they may pursue multiple options at the same time; however, they maintain a focus on the customers needs and wants.

Psychological traits of development personnel

There are obvious differences between basic researchers and those involved in product development. For the most part, basic scientists seek fundamental discoveries and achievements are measured by the number and quality of published papers and personnel reputation in the scientific community. Support is garnered from research grants. On the other hand, development personnel may carry on some basic research, but for the most part are interested in products, processes, and services that can be manufactured, sold, delivered and serviced [1]. Their achievements are measured by patents and, because they need to protect proprietary information, publications are not primary mechanisms for advancing their reputations. They receive financial compensation instead and do not compete for grant support. Since they are motivated to provide commercial products, the direction of their research may change rapidly to fulfil customer needs.

Management of developmental personnel

Scientists respect leaders in their field. Likewise, good managers are also respected for their professionalism. It is incumbent upon a director of development to become proficient in management skills and impart to their staff an understanding of the social benefits of technological transfer, including a need for fiscal responsibility. The driving force for development includes a vision of the future and well defined goals.

Factors that provide the impetus for development programs can be divided into eight categories: 1) products driven, 2) markets served, 3) return/profit, 4) technology-driven, 5) low-cost production capabilities, 6) operating capabilities, 7) method of distribution/sales, and 8) natural resources.

Management is responsible for defining vision: The focus of future development, the scope of products and markets that will be considered, and the emphasis on priorities for the future. If the products offered by a company provide the driving force for new ventures, organization must define the characteristics of its products and develop new ones that fit those characteristics. If the driving force is defined by the market that is served, the organization's growth is centered on its relationships with the markets or customers it serves and fulfilment of their needs. Such organizations usually have strong and well-defined relationships with their customers. If the driving force is return/profit, then the organization strives to keep businesses or products that return a profit.

For the most part blood centers are driven by a "products-offered" or "market-served" force. Hence, future development aims at developing new products or new markets. An example of how vision and driving force interact is the development of Clinical Laboratories at the Blood Center of Southeastern

Wisconsin. The platelet antibody laboratory is a direct outgrowth of a basic science interest in platelet immunology. The regional hemostasis laboratory was a direct outgrowth of investigators' interests in von Willebrand factor and protein C. The laboratories were initiated as a result of requests for laboratory tests from clinicians and hospitals within and beyond the region served by the center. Clearly, a combination of a products-driven and market-service approach to development of basic research investigations led to development of specialty laboratories.

Creation of a conducive milieu for development

The establishment of a conducive milieu for development personnel is analogous to that for basic research. It begins with top management in defining a vision for the future, acquisition of managers with professional skills and setting the stage for defining benefits of research to patients, clinicians, etc.

Perhaps most important is the recognition of the requirement that developmental scientists must interact continuously with basic researchers. They must be able to identify and implement new findings quickly. This is one of the outstanding lessons of the Bell Laboratories System. It houses both basic and applied engineering scientists. Without this type of constant interaction, basic research might be conducted in a vacuum and opportunities for technology transfer may be missed. Likewise, without applied scientists, exciting innovations might be retained within a laboratory's walls.

Benefits of research and development programs at blood centers

In today's atmosphere of continuous quality improvement, it may not be apparent that a blood center research program requires justification or an explanation of its benefits. Perhaps foremost, research serves as an entrée to development: The lightning rod for new technology. A strong research program fulfils a blood center's role in advancing knowledge about blood banking, immunohematology and transfusion medicine. It serves an organizational need in keeping the center informed of new medical and technical development. Other benefits that affect the internal operations of the blood center include interaction with a center's educational programs, working with a center's laboratories to assure implementation of new developments, and an overall enhancement of the staff's self-image because they are employed at a "cutting edge" organization, (personal communication Richard H. Aster).

From the point of view of a blood center's relationship with the external environment, a successful research program enhances its visibility in the community and facilitates its interaction with local and regional academic institutions. Both of these "benefits" are in reality quite substantial. There is also transferability of this positive image to a center's service and educational commitments. Good relationships with academic institutions are critical since these institutions are usually influential in community affairs.

Risks of a research and development program to a blood center

The major risk posed to a blood center by research and development programs is a loss of focus from the main service commitment of collecting, processing and distributing blood and components. This may occur as a result of the extensive time commitment required on behalf of top management. It may also occur because the need for entrepreneurial spirit and commercial development conflicts with a center's altruistically-based service requirements. Space and developmental costs are a potent financial threat if outside funding sources are insufficient to cover direct and indirect research costs. Fear of being contaminated by "commercialization" can lead to the loss of superior academic talent and a possible loss of autonomy in research initiatives. As a result, management must maintain constant vigilance to prevent this. In addition, there are inevitable conflicts between researchers and those involved in development. The goals, performance evaluations, and rewards of the groups are different. A similar problem occurs between research and operations staff when personnel from these areas work in close proximity. Persons involved in nursing, donor drawing, blood processing, component preparation, etc., are expected to fit into the organizational mold whereas researchers are accustomed to autonomy and, not infrequently, flaunt authority.

Conclusion

Blood center research and development programs, if properly managed, add significantly to a center's prestige, talent base and ability to contribute to acquisition to new knowledge. In turn, recruitment of sufficient numbers of new investigators is facilitated. If properly chosen, they will work together to form a critical mass that builds on itself. This in turn spawns applications that impact directly on patients and clinicians. The net result is growth in service opportunities, enhancement of the center's programs and increased revenues. With proper "vision" from top management, blood centers provide an ideal environment for research and development programs.

References

1. Montague MJ. A university-industry partnership approach to technology transfer. Product and Process Innovation 1991;1:19-23.
2. The American Red Cross. The American Red Cross biomedical research and development report, Rockville MD, 1989.
3. Montgomery RR. Personal communication.
4. Drucker PF. The 10 rules of effective research. Wall Street Journal 1989, May 30.
5. Ross IM. AT&T Bell Laboratories: Information technology. In: Carnegie Institute of Washington Address, 1991:1-8.
6. Todd KB. A capsule history of the Bell System – compiled and edited from previously published material.
7. Bylinsky G. Technology: The new look at American's top lab. Fortune 1988 [reprint].

122

8.Gilhooly D. A mission from AT&T. Telecommunications 1988 [reprint].

9.AT&T Bell Laboratories. Lab Notes: Photons, microchips, and software: Bell Labs zeros in on the year 2000. June, 1991.

10.Blood Center of Southeastern Wisconsin. Milwaukee, WI. Annual Report, 1991.

11.New York Blood Center. New York, NY. Annual Report, 1989-90.

12.Puget Sound Blood Program. Seattle, WA. Annual Report, 1988/1989.

13.Puget Sound Blood Program. Seattle, WA. Annual Report. 1990.

14.Reeves ET. The management of scientific and technical personnel [unpublished].

15.Quinn JB. Managing innovation: Controlled chaos. Harvard Business Review. Boston, MA, May/June 1986.

SPECIALIZATION IN TRANSFUSION MEDICINE BY UNDER- AND POSTGRADUATE TRAINING

G. Matthes, E. Richter

Introduction

This paper focuses on the problems of undergraduate training in transfusion medicine. Transfusion medicine started more than 50 years ago as blood banking and became now a medical discipline, with own theoretical and practical fundaments. Recently, M.A. Blajchman described this new discipline [1]: "Transfusion medicine is that multidisciplinary branch of medicine that focuses on all the available medical, scientific, and technical information applicable to this speciality for the benefit of patients receiving blood products or related materials produced by biotechnology. Those engaged in the practice of transfusion medicine have the responsibility of integrating the various concepts, techniques, and other elements of relevant knowledge from contributing disciplines such as blood banking, immunohematology, infectious diseases, immunology, transplantation biology, genetics, protein chemistry, molecular and cell biology, clinical medicine, laboratory sciences, epidemiology, microbiology, and virology. Issues relating to the recruitment of donors and the collection of whole blood and blood components, such as the psychology of the motivation of donors, are also germane, as are legal and ethical questions associated with the collection and the clinical use of blood products.

Those engaged in transfusion medicine should also be involved in education and research relevant to the speciality. Curricular goals for the teaching of transfusion medicine have been outlined recently as have relevant research opportunities."

Undergraduate training in transfusion medicine

In contrast to other relatively new medical disciplines (like clinical pharmacology) there is no compulsory or special undergraduate training of medical students in most universities in Europe [2]. But only the teaching of students in transfusion medicine provides knowledge in this field for all future physicians (and more than 50% of all physicians are involved in transfusion problems at all).

Table 1. Curriculum of medical students for the 3rd academic year at Humboldt University in Berlin; School of Medicine (Charité), Humboldt University of Berlin, (extract).

Subject	Total hours	Hours per week per term			
		Lect.	Tut.	Class	Pract.
3rd Academic year *(1st and 2nd clinical term)*					
Internal medicine	180	2	2	4	4
Surgery	60	1	1	1	1
Pathology	168	4	2	3	2
Pathophysiology	64	3	–	1	–
Clinical chemistry	76	2	1	1	1
Microbiology	79	1	1	1	1.5
Immunology	48	2	–	1	–
Pharmacology	120	2	2	2	2
History of medicine	28	–	1.75	–	0.25
Biostatistics	28	–	1	–	1
Transfusion medicine	16	0.75	–	–	0.25
Oncology	10	–	0.75	–	–

Since 1978 at the Medical School (Charité) at the Humboldt University in Berlin a regular teaching program for medical students in transfusion medicine is included in the student's curriculum offered by the Institute of Transfusion Medicine where a professorship of transfusion medicine exists since 1985.

The teaching program involves a total of 18 lessons for students in their third academic year (Table 1). The teaching program in transfusion medicine consists of lectures, tutorial classes and practical training. Figure 1 shows the main points of the teaching program in transfusion medicine. The twelve lectures deal with fundamental aspects of transfusion medicine (history of blood transfusion; organization of the transfusion service; guidelines for blood transfusion; medical, social, and legal aspects of blood donation), with transfusion immunology (nomenclature; ABO- and Rhesus-system; further clinically important blood group systems; pretransfusion serology; type-screen-and-hold-systems; antibody screening and detection; HLA-, granulocyte- and platelet specific systems; diagnosis and prophylaxis of sensibilization as a result of transfusion of blood and blood components), with fundamental aspects of blood component preparation (medical and logistic aspects; hemapheresis procedures; separation and preservation of blood cells; indication and contraindication of the application of blood and blood components; transmission of infectious diseases by blood products; fractionation and isolation of blood and blood components; artificial blood substitutes), with aspects of clinical transfusion therapy

Lectures (12 hours)
- Fundamentals of transfusion medicine   2 hours
- Transfusion immunology   4 hours
- Fundamentals of blood component preparation   2 hours
- Transfusion therapy   4 hours

Practical training (4 hours)
- Blood group typing (ABO- and Rhesus-typing)
- Compatibility testing (incl. AHG)
- Bed-side-test

Figure 1. Main fields of the training program in the special field of transfusion medicine at Humboldt University in Berlin.

- Obligation
- Binding character of the training program
- Sole responsibility and guidance by specialists
- Temporal bounds
- Local bounds
- Evidence of attainments

Figure 2. Elements of further education to qualify as a specialist in transfusion medicine.

(pathophysiology of blood loss and transfusion; hemotherapy of blood loss in surgery, in internal medicine, paediatrics, and oncology; hemotherapy of plasmatic disorders; problems of emergency and massive transfusion; preparative and therapeutic cyt- and plasmapheresis; therapy of transfusion reactions, autologous transfusion concepts).

The topics of teaching in transfusion medicine were fixed after discussions with lectures in physiology, immunology, hematology, clinical chemistry, surgery, and microbiology in order to prevent overlapping of teaching contents.

Teaching in transfusion medicine includes both theoretical and practical teaching. The lecturers are completed by a two-hour tutorial class and a four hour practical training in order to repeat and consolidate basic knowledge in transfusion medicine. In this practical training every student exercises a complete blood group typing (ABO-, Rhesus-), a crossmatch test, AHG- and a bed-side-test. At the end of the teaching period the students have to pass an examination in the frame of practical training.

Since 1978 more than 5,000 students passed this training in transfusion medicine (350 students per year). In 1988 we tried to evaluate the efficiency of this teaching program by means of a multiple-choice-test. A total of 20 questions had to be answered by the students in their last academic year as well as in their first clinical year as physician. As a result of this evaluation we could see that the knowledge in the field of transfusion medicine increased over the last years. As an example in 1980 only 25% of the students answered more than half of all questions with marks better than two (60% of question right), in 1988 more than 60% of all students [3]. It is of special interest that the students accept this form of teaching in transfusion medicine and understand the importance of this teaching concept for their medical education.

Postgraduate training in transfusion medicine

Specialists in transfusion medicine have been trained in Berlin since 1962 [5]. This further education to qualify as a specialist is provided by standards (coordinated by an expert Commission for Transfusion Medicine which also holds the final colloquia by the end of the specialized further education). Figure2 shows the elements of this postgraduate education. The training program comprises the goal, theoretical and practical subject matters, instructions of the course of further education, and the different forms of testing the trainee's attainments.

The lifelong postgraduate education in transfusion medicine for maintaining professional capability is based on different elements. Beside the individual private readings, special importance is attached in this connection to the national and international Transfusion Medicine Societies. Since the contact between colleagues is attributed a high rank to within the special branch [4], training courses and group auditing on selected topics (e.g. the diagnosis of transfusion-serological problem cases, histocompatibility testing for transfusions and transplantations, cryopreservation of blood cells, clinical transfusion medicine, quality control, cyt- and plasmapheresis) are organized which should be attended by each specialist once every five years.

The Institute of Transfusion Medicine offers individual and group auditing in the field of clinical transfusion medicine, concepts in autologous transfusion, preparation and separation of blood cells, strategies for pretransfusion serology, tissue banking of allo- and xenografts, cryopreservation of blood cells and tissues.

References

1. Blajchman MA. Defining transfusion medicine (editorial). Transfusion Medicine Reviews 1990;4:169.
2. Rossi U, Cash JD (eds). Teaching in transfusion medicine. Proceedings of the First SIITS-AICT Symposium for European Cooperation, Cernobbio, October 1990.
3. Freistedt B. Untersuchung zur Ausbildung von Medizinstudenten im Fach Transfusionsmedizin. Abschlußarbeit im postgradualen Studium Hochschulpädagogik, Humboldt-Universität zu Berlin, 1988.

4. Matthes G. Fortbildung durch Fachliteratur – Ergebnisse einer Befragung von Fachärzten für Blutspende- und Transfusionswezen. Zärtzl Fortbildung (Jena) 1983;77: 899-90.
5. Matthes G. Under- and postgraduate education in the field of Transfusion Medicine in the German Democratic Republic. In: Castelli D, Genatet B, Habibi B, Nydegger UE (eds). Transfusion in Europe. Arnette SA, Paris 1990:283-5.

DISCUSSION

B. Habibi, P.C. Das

P.C. Das (Groningen, NL): There is difference of attitude of mind involved in the practice of Transfusion Medicine, for example in the use of irradiated blood products. This attitude is derived from the institutional information system. But where is the knowledge out of this information and where is the wisdom that is lying behind this knowledge. Caring is as important as curing. It is as important to sustain the life, where there is so little left in acutely ill patients in emergency and surgery. In our educational process in the Western culture we get tools like chisels and hammers, like apheresis leukocyte poor blood. But what you do with it and what you make out of it, is up to us.

C.Th. Smit Sibinga: Talking about Transfusion Medicine, there is still a lot of confusion. In a recent consultation in Geneva to the GBSI program of the World Health Organization, we came to the following description of what Transfusion Medicine actually should be. It said that "Transfusion Medicine is that part of the health care system which undertakes the appropriate provision and the use of blood resources". Then comes the part where I think most of the confusion is in, Transfusion Practice which is different from Transfusion Medicine; "if we make the working assumption that Transfusion Practice is that collective activity which links the donor with the patient, then it follows that Transfusion Medicine occupies those areas in which it is deemed important or even essential that a medical practitioner contributes to this bridging process". I think that we should be aware of these two inter-related aspects: The Transfusion Practice and the Transfusion Medicine as such. I think this is at least part of the confusion and therefore the fiction. Echoing what Dr. Gibbs was presenting, we also recognize that the teaching and the training must be directed to a safe and efficient performance. The three major areas, which Dr. Gibbs has presented, are indeed the motivation, recruitment and retention of blood donors, but also the processing and the testing which includes collection, laboratory testing, preparation of blood products, GMP being a very important aspect. Then there are the storage and the distribution and the appropriate clinical use of blood and blood components. Additionally, as Dr. Gibbs has listed as point four is the focusing on the management, the administrative aspects. Not to forget also is technical maintenance, an important aspect which we should pay attention to. So, I think here we have the scope of what we are talking about.

C.F. Högman: I would just like to make a comment on Dr. Smit Sibinga's paper about inspection. I recall when we started what we could call inspection, although we did call it consultation and education. We served a number of small hospital blood banks, because they quite often do not have the expertise in the own hospital. They really need supervision and education. At the beginning we were met with suspicion and not all were particularly interested to show what they were doing or really to discuss. But after some time we could set up some mutual trust, which I would say is very important. As soon as they realized that we were there to help and actually could provide something, then it went so much better. Actually we could then achieve what we had as goal namely uniform standards as a very important improvement really of the service within our region. This was instituted regionally and my own view is that it might be easier to have it regionally, because it is easier then also to have a continuous personal contact between the inspector and those being inspected.

C.Th. Smit Sibinga: I think that is a valuable addition to the same mechanism, because what you are actually saying is that you provide the help, you get the provision for how to get to a better and safer and more effective practice and come gradually to some type of standard.

T.F. Zuck: Maybe a contrary view of the definition of Transfusion Medicine may be in order. I really cannot speak for Europe, but I can speak for what has happened in the United States. The kinds of skills that are needed to engineer shop floors, to learn how to keep batch records, to learn how to set up auditing procedures, to learn how to detect error prior to the time error effects the outcome are skills and technologies that we as physicians are hopelessly inadequate in. I think if we as physicians in Transfusion Medicine want to say we are going to learn those skills then that is fine, but to wring our hands and say that Federal Government is practising medicine, which is terrible, to me is not really relevant. I think Transfusion Medicine starts when we make decisions about therapy for patients.

Today I think the manufacturing of blood and blood components with zero lot-to-lot variation and with good manufacturing practices according to the FDA, with the 200 Series of rigid, stringent types of process controls is needed in Transfusion Medicine. However, there is a whole group of professionals that does not know how to do that. We need to have a discussion about the complications in Transfusion Medicine, because we are just looking at the problem with two sets of eyes very differently.

C.Th. Smit Sibinga: Is that a comment, is it a fiction or a faction.

T.F. Zuck: The fact that in the United States we are going to be held to comply with the standards of the 200 Series of Title 21 is a fact, it is not a fiction; the FDA has made that decision. For those who do not know what that means, in the United States we have been regulated on what we called the 600 Series,[1] which are the more permissive biological standards. The standards of the 200 Series of Title 21 are much more rigorous, including the GMP procedures. Dr. Cash just told me that in Scotland end-lot testing is done on the pools and if hepatitis is found, the whole lot made from that pool goes out. That is new in terms of how people are approaching lot-to-lot variation. If we are going to include those principles in Transfusion Medicine and claim hold to it, we have to learn engineering and pharmaceutical techniques.

D. Goldfinger: Maybe I can make a comment. Dr. Zuck, the fact is that I am right and the fiction is that you are right. I think that what you are really saying is no different from what I said. Perhaps an analogy is in the moral of infectious disease. There are specialists in infectious disease who treat patients, then there are manufacturers of pharmaceuticals, of antibiotics for example. To a large extent these areas of expertise are very separate and so I would agree with you that an infectious disease specialist probably has little knowledge and certainly little capability of running a pharmaceutical manufacturing company. We in blood banking are expected to have both of these kinds of expertise and perhaps that is unfortunate. I think a lot of very fine blood bankers in the last couple of years have gotten into a lot of trouble because they are excellent Transfusion Medicine specialists and were denigrated to some extent for their inability to manage something that they were never asked to do before in the way they are asked to do it now by following these very strict rules in regulations. So, in order for this specialty to survive the way we would like to see it namely as a very high class operation, we do need to separate to some extent the functions of those involved in the manufacturing process and those involved in the delivery of care to patients. As Dr. Menitove pointed out perhaps another segment in which there can certainly be participation of the same individuals is in the research and development sector which again is to some extent separate when we look at the management of infectious disease.

P.C. Das: Dr. Urbaniak, in your presentation there was quite a lovely concept of continuous education and Prof. Matthes had produced what could be taught at undergraduate level. How could you see this is being developed in your system?

S.J. Urbaniak (Aberdeen, Scotland): That is a major topic in its own right. I think I did mention that there is an entire book of presentations on the contents of Transfusion Medicine training programs, which will shortly be available. I have addressed myself only to the concept of assessing fitness to practice as

1.   Code of Federal Regulations.

you define it. I did not set myself the task of defining what that fitness should be and what the content of the training program should be. That is a very important major topic, but I did not set out to address that.

P.C. Das: I favour continuous research as presented by Dr. Menitove. How do you see the research and development aspects in the continuous education in Transfusion Medicine, what role would it play in your idea?

S.J. Urbaniak: Well, let me say that the critical concept is not a matter of training in the didactic sense of presenting training programs. It is a mechanism of thought. It is an approach to the subject in terms of how in a sense you place your own activities; how you assess your own standards against others. The critical aspect is to determine what the standard should be. That is where so much of the fiction comes in many respects; the fiction is that many of the standards are set somewhat arbitrarily. The point I make is that particularly in transfusion support it is not to assess who is right and who is wrong, but what is best.

J.E. Menitove: Just a follow-up. I do not see where we can wear separate hats at different times; there are service commitments that we have to fulfil, there are educational aspects that we want to fulfil and some centres are lucky enough to be involved in research and development. I think the art is mixing it together, including what Dr. Zuck has said. There is also a large element of education in terms of learning what the 200 Series is and how it applies to what we do. I think that people involved in senior management need to educate the profession about what that means. So, I see it all in a continuum.

B. Habibi: I like to return back to the very important question of Dr. Zuck. If I understood correctly, you are advocating the dissociation of the two great poles, provision from care. That in my sense is a bit restrictive and is keeping with the current trend we heard about, giving to the preparation and the provision some pharmaceutical identity and to confine the definition of Transfusion Medicine. My impression is that blood transfusion is unique and that it is a combination of multiple boxes linking the donor to the recipient. Why not putting all those links of the chain within the same activity? That is the essence of my definition of Transfusion Medicine, because otherwise it will be very difficult to manage the whole system and to keep the link between the donor and the recipient.

T.F. Zuck: Dr. Habibi, I do not disagree at all. I was addressing an education point and tried to comment on Smit Sibinga's definition. What I was trying to say is, that if we are going to treat Transfusion Medicine with all the flexibility of a physician being captain of his ship having all discretion that he desires in practising medicine, it will be essentially the way we run blood centres. What I was really trying to point out is that we no longer can do that. If we are going to say Transfusion Medicine embraces all we do in a blood centre then physicians or anyone that runs a blood centre has to learn a whole new discipline, process engineering, design flow, and the like. So, what we hear so much is that there is too much regulation. What I am saying is we have to take the New York Blood Centre model: Have a pharmaceutical expert run the blood operations and have a respected internationally known physician run the clinical application side of Transfusion Medicine. Most of us have to embody most of those skills in the person responsible who is a physician. This means, we have to learn process engineering, shop floor design, Title 200, etc. On the whole we have to educate ourselves or we will fail to meet the public expectations and the expectations of the regulating authorities.

J.D. Cash: I think we do not have the answers to many of these questions, however, I think one of the great values of this meeting here in Groningen are these debates. There was a debate about Transfusion Medicine in the early 1980s. Here we are in the 1990s and the debate is starting again. I can see it going on and on and on and I welcome this. I would make a small point on the infectious diseases model referred to by Dr. Goldfinger. Medical practitioners play a critical role in the pharmaceutical industry. So critical is this role that in Europe there is a separate medical specialty for doctors in the pharmaceutical industry. They have their own training programs and professional examinations. These doctors do not seem to be over-concerned with the principles of flexibility to practise. The debate will continue as to how much Transfusion Medicine will contribute to Transfusion Practice, but I believe we would be well advised to retain that tradition of flexibility held so dearly by the medical profession. Thus we should embrace the challenges of good manufacturing practice and the Series 200. But at the same time we need to look carefully at our work at the clinical interface. This is not always quite what we imagine it to be.

P.C. Das: The point that Dr. Goldfinger brought up was the fact that in one hand we are doing our best to put all the rules and regulations in place, and here comes the patient with what I call the little life left worth saving in the operation theatre in emergency which may require going over the so-called standards. How does one solve this dilemma as a physician?

J.D. Cash: It is important that we appreciate that our American colleagues are currently distracted with the prospect of persecution by lawyers. I feel sorry for them, and recognize that they seek to build walls and castles to defend themselves. What Dr. Goldfinger is emphasizing is that some of these walls and castles are not in our patients' interest. How right he is! We are very fortunate in Europe, for we can consider the development of Transfusion Medicine without the spectre of undue pressure from the legal profession.

C.Th. Smit Sibinga: Just a quick comment, Dr. Zuck; I can feel your worries, on the other hand I think, if we agree on the fact that Transfusion Medicine as a multidisciplinary field covers all what is between the donor and the patient, there should not be any fear for comprehending more information, more technology when you want to be in the lead. That is a natural development; we have gone into automation, we have gone into medical sociology. We heard a marvellous presentation of Mr. Los on a field, which we have to comprehend also. Biotechnology has entered Transfusion Medicine, has even firmly found its place in Transfusion Medicine. That does not necessarily mean that we all need to be biotechnical engineers. You need not be an explicit expert in the details of each of these fields. Yet, you have to comprehend these aspects and these are natural developments. I do not see what is wrong with that. There is room for all these disciplines within Transfusion Medicine as I stated before.

T.F. Zuck: I fully agree with you and with what Dr. Habibi said. I was trying to address the educational point, because this is an educational forum. Transfusion Medicine is so different and the disciplines we have to embrace are demanding, somewhat like the Japanese autoindustry technologies. What I am saying is that for when we are going to embrace this, than we in fact must be very serious about how we educate ourselves in these skills. We cannot reduce lot-to-lot variations without these skills.

W.N. Gibbs: Prof. Matthes, has there been any attempt to measure the application of training. You spoke about enough multiple-choice questions for people who have done the undergraduate training program, but what really matters in the end is how it is applied in practice. I also question the wisdom of separating the training of undergraduates in Transfusion Medicine or applied Transfusion Medicine from other disciplines because of its relationship with other disciplines. I think there should be a closer relationship and there should not be an attempt at separation at such an early stage. The last point concerns the education of physicians. We heard about those early after graduation, but what happens later on about continuity of education of physicians and the appropriate use of blood and blood components.

G. Matthes (Berlin, FRG): Dr. Gibbs, concerning your first question how to evaluate the efficiency of a training program, we have experience with multiple-choice tests. Every two years we gave the same questions to students who passed this training program three or four years before. So we could compare the results, the answers and it was not difficult to estimate the efficiency among the students. A problem is the postgraduate training of young physicians with different knowledge in Transfusion Medicine, because in our hospital are working not only physicians that graduated from the Medical School Charité, but also from other universities. There is great difference between the universities in the level of undergraduate medical training.

The second question – education and the teaching of Transfusion Medicine for physicians who are not specialists in Transfusion Medicine. I think we should draw more attention to this point, because most physicians have their knowledge only by contact with colleagues, by literature, by reading a publication or by their own experience. What we really need is a continuous education, continuous teaching in Transfusion Medicine because it is a very small, very specialized medical discipline. So we can teach a basic knowledge in Transfusion Medicine on one hand and on the other hand we will be able to control an optimal usage of blood and blood components.

Regarding your third question; I agree with you, we need a life-long education in Transfusion Medicine also for experienced physicians to maintain their professional capability in the field of Transfusion Medicine. This is not only true for the specialists in Transfusion Medicine, but also for the people working in surgery, anesthesiology and other medical fields. We should pay more attention to this life-long postgraduate training in Transfusion Medicine by training courses or group auditings.

B. Habibi: Mr. Los, I was impressed by the data you showed. The question I would like to ask is how do you use your data and your experience? How do you exploit them, what kind of recommendations would you like to make in order to go further to implement your results and conclusions?

A.P.M. Los (Groningen, NL): I would like to emphasize that the starting point is sound demographics of general population and donor population. I do realize that registers of demographic data are not implemented in all countries, yet. So, I think that before talking about reaching the community we should have good data on the community that is to be reached. It may be very basic, but basic demographics are the starting point. What I showed consisted of a lot of data management; data management on the demographics of the general population that we have access to from the Central Bureau of Statistics in our country. The second point is the adjustment of the data from our donors. Comparing both populations would lead to a lot of data management before you can even compare. We developed standard procedures for managing data available from the general population and donor population. I would like to recommend general implementation of the same method for registration; and more important, looking for possibilities for mutual exchange between blood centres and availability of these anonymized data, so you can have more possibilities for comparing.

J.D. Cash: Mr. Los, I was interested in your conclusion that the young women in Groningen are "easy come, easy go". Are you aware of any other institutions in which similar demographic work is under way and whether this view of young women in the context of blood transfusion, is specific to Groningen or has a more general application?

A.P.M. Los: Well, I think that the demographics of donor populations have been subject to many studies. However, what we often see in these studies is the demographics of the population at a specific moment, which could result in observed differences in the age distribution of the male and female donor population, but does not differentiate between those who come and those who go or resign. What we have done is looking at the male and female first-time donor population and looking at the male and female resigned donor population, and the length of the male and female donor career over the period from 1983 until 1989. In a way we looked more into the dynamics of the donor population. Thus, what we are eager to do in the future is, to study the donor population as a "box" with an input and an output speaking in terms of system theory. Going further, you could even make a computer model of the donor population and just manipulate what is coming in and what is going out. This would allow to study how the donor population is developing in the future. Returning to the results of our donor demographics, you have seen there is a lot of input from the younger population, specifically from the younger female population. What you also see is a lot of output from the younger female population, resulting in the differences in the demographic composition of the female and the male donor population. If you wonder whether this is the case only in Groningen, then similar studies on donor demographics and the dynamics of the donor population in other areas could give the answer.

H.H. Gunson (Manchester, UK): We have carried out in England a demographic study of donors. I was very interested to see your results, because we have a mirror of many of your findings in the study we have done which will be presented in Prague.[1] One significant fact was that it was not difficult to motivate people to become donors. Social conscience and the fact that they are helping someone else or a member of the family who had received a blood transfusion were the main motivating factors. However, what staggered us in the interviews, that were carried out with over 7000 members of the general public who were randomly chosen was that 28% of them had at some time donated blood and currently we have 4% of the population on our donor panels. That means that although some of these may have been lost through medical illness, somehow due to disenchantment we had a large number of the people in the general population who had stopped donating blood. Protection of our service means that we have to prevent the loss of donors, and donor retention seems to me the major aspect on which we have to concentrate for the future.

A.P.M. Los: Well, I certainly agree and I hope that in my presentation it was clear that retention of donors is one of the major points.

Hu Ching-li: If I may take just a few minutes. I think I should congratulate Mr. Los who did such a kind of study, because we did a lot of studies on the medical sciences, but very few on the social and the behaviourial sciences. So, I think this is an important area we have to also continue because we know

1.   3rd. Congress of the European Division of the ISBT, Prague, October 1991.

that it is very easy to motivate the donors, but how to maintain these donors who can keep on coming. We want to have a further step to find the solution. To follow Dr. Cash who said "The young women are easy come and easy go". Can we get them "Easy coming and not so easy go" and retain them as a donor? So, what is the solution for this?

A.P.M. Los: Well, I wish I had a solution to this problem. One can try to investigate the reasons for resigning. I think that the majority of the resignations in the younger donor population, female donor population, is without known specific reason. They just stay away, they quit and we do not know why. We just finished our study on demographics which lasted two years. To implement the results, we plan to do exit interviews, exit questionnaires, just to know why they leave and particularly why they leave so quickly.

G.A. van Voolen (Jamesville, NY, USA): I would like to make a comment. I think that if we had a psychologist involved then that would make a significant difference in finding out why people want to stay away, once they do stay away. Also this would be good for how to get people to be involved. Furthermore, an advertiser or a marketing specialist would also be very useful to retain for these purposes.

U. Rossi: Don't you think that the suspensions for pregnancies could easily explain this difference in behaviour between young men and young women.

A.P.M. Los: Suspension for pregnancies could certainly explain a part of the difference in behaviour between young male and female donors. Of course, we have also analyzed the known reasons, including pregnancies, why female donors do resign compared to male donors; there are many differences in that sort of reasons. However, I must stress again, that there is a substantial group of donors from which we do not know the reasons why they quit. Only further research in this specific group of donors can give answers on the questions of the origin of the differences.

M. Rustam: Dr. Gibbs, you showed that training programs organized by WHO started in 1978. But there was a training course many years before in 1967 and 1968 organized by WHO in Budapest. There were participants from twelve countries. It was a six months course, divided into two parts. The first part were lectures in the morning and practical laboratory work in the afternoon, followed by on the job training in different blood centres. I was one of the participants at the time and I think this course was very useful. My question is, why such a course does not exist anymore?

W.N. Gibbs: Well, first of all let me thank you for letting me know about that. The main reason in fact why that kind of course has not taken place more often, is a lack of funding, which is one of the problems we face. In general people do not regard this as a priority and we are working on this to try to correct that kind of problem.

IV. HISTORICAL ASPECTS AND FUTURE PERSPECTIVES

TRANSFUSION MEDICINE: HISTORICAL OVERVIEW
The Eras of Serology, Component Production and Fractionation

C.F. Högman

Introduction

Although blood transfusions had been given already in the 17th century, it was not until Karl Landsteiner had discovered the blood groups in 1900-1901 that a reasonably safe transfer of blood from one person to another could be performed. The second important part in the foundation of transfusion medicine was the finding that citrate was a potent inhibitor of blood coagulation with very low toxicity in humans. A. Hustin, L. Agote, R. Lewisohn and R. Weil independently were investigating several aspects of citrate during the years before and at the time of the First World War [1,p.39]. Citrated blood was used during this war but otherwise direct transfusion from donor to recipient was the most common route of transfusion in the 20-year period before the Second World War.

The real birth of transfusion medicine in a modern sense took place during the second world war when the great importance of blood transfusion in the treatment of hemorrhagic shock was more widely recognized. The discovery of the Rh blood groups by Levine and Stetson (1939) and Landsteiner and Wiener (1940) [2,p.156], as well as new techniques to demonstrate the binding of IgG class antibodies – in those days called incomplete or blocking antibodies – to red cells, contributed strongly to the safety of allogeneic transfusion. The rediscovery of the antiglobulin technique of C. Moreschi (1908) made by R. Coombs, R. Race, and A. Mourant (1945) had an enormous impact on blood group serology [2,p.409].

Another important discovery was made by Loutit and Mollison (1943) demonstrating that the red cells, needing glucose for refrigerator temperature storage, were better kept at a slightly acid rather than a neutral pH. The acidity of the anticoagulant was originally applied to avoid caramelization of the glucose during autoclaving [2,p.58]; in fact it does counteract an alkaline pH in the red cell at 4°C. Rapoport's studies published in 1947 in a special issue of J Clin Invest [see 1] indicated that a maintained red cell viability was dependent on a reasonably well maintained erythrocyte adenosine triphosphate (ATP) concentration. This finding was later confirmed and extended by others and had

Table 1. The foundation of Transfusion Medicine.

1900	K. Landsteiner: Discovery of the blood groups
1914	A. Hustin, L. Agote, R. Lewisohn, R. Weil: Citrate is a suitable anticoagulant with low toxicity
First World War	Citrated blood is used in blood transfusion
1920–1940	Blood transfusions uncommon. Mostly direct transfer from donor to recipient
1939	P. Levine, R. Stetson: Immunological mechanism as the cause of Hemolytic Disease of the Newborn (HDN)
1940	K. Landsteiner, A. Wiener: Discovery of the Rh blood groups by immunizing rabbits and guinea pigs with red cells from Rhesus macacus monkeys
1943	J. Loutit, P. Mollison: ACD solution makes storage of red cells possible
1945	R. Coombs, R. Race, A. Mourant: The birth of modern blood group serology
1947	S. Rapoport: Red cell viability related to maintenance of ATP

a great importance for the improvement of the storage conditions for red cells. The major steps in the development described above are summarized in Table 1.

The era of blood group serology – the 1950s (summarized in Table 2)

Subsequent to the first and fundamental discoveries before and during the 1940s, the decennium of the 1950s can be said to be that of blood group serology. The mapping of the red cell blood groups was largely extended and blood group serology became a standard procedure in pre-transfusion testing. New surgical techniques, thoracic surgery in particular, should not have been possible without the availability of donor blood for transfusion. Well organized blood trans-

Table 2. The era of blood group serology - the 1950s.

1950	F. Allen, L. Diamond and others: Exchange transfusion effective treatment of Hemolytic Disease of the Newborn (HDN)
1945–	R. Ceppellini, M. Cutbusch & P. Mollison, P. Levine, A. Mourant, R. Race & R. Sanger, R. Rosenfield, C. Salmon, J. van Loghem, A. Wiener and others: Blood group serology dominates the scientific discussion
1948–	W. Morgan, W. Watkins, E. Kabat: The birth of blood group chemistry
1945–	Blood transfusion services, often founded in the late 1940s, become established; emphasis on blood donor recruitment

fusion services became a necessity as well as active blood donor recruitment. The mechanisms of hemolytic disease of the newborn, as first indicated by Levine and Stetson, was a rapid destruction of the fetus/ infant's red cells due to passively transferred maternal antibodies.

Diamond in 1947 [3] introduced exchange transfusion as a much more effective way of treatment than transfusion alone. The purpose was to remove 1) the antibody-coated red cells; and 2) the bilirubin. This soon became accepted as the method of choice. Allen, Diamond, and Vaughan [4] in 1950 showed that kernicterus could be prevented. In order to find the mothers whose fetuses were threatened, general ante-natal Rh grouping was instituted of all pregnant women with subsequent screening for Rh antibodies in those found Rh negative.

This was also the decade when the chemical nature of the blood groups and the way they were inherited started to be clarified due to the elegant studies of W. Morgan, W. Watkins, E. Kabat and others. It became clear that the genes governed the synthesis of transferases which transform basic substances into shapes that could initiate the formation and recognition of specific antibodies. This biochemical work made the connection between the ABO and Lewis blood groups and the secretor/non-secretor status understandable.

The era of immunology – the 1960s (summarized in Table 3)

For a long time immunology had been equivalent to serology. In the early 1960s two types of lymphocytes, the B and T cells, were discovered, as well as their roles in humoral and cellular immune reactions, respectively. This changed the perspective and the interest was much focused on cellular immunology and the mechanism for the specificity of the immune system.

Already in 1953 J. Dausset had found the first leukocyte alloantibodies and later recognized the first leukocyte blood group called Mac. In the 1960s extensive studies of the blood groups of lymphocytes were carried out. probably the possibility to use an extreme micro-technique, first introduced by Terasaki

Table 3. The era of immunology – the 1960s.

1962	Discovery of B and T lymphocytes; humoral and cellular immunity
1953–	J. Dausset: Leukocyte alloantigens
1966–	B. Bain, F. Bach, F. Kissmeyer-Nielsen, R. Payne, J. van Rood, P. Terasaki and others: Discovery of the HLA system
1970s	The clinical importance of the HLA system in organ and bone marrow transplantation is established
1970s	E.D. Thomas and others: Demonstration of the usefulness of bone marrow transplantation in hematological aplasia and malignancies
1973	G. Opelz, P. Terasaki and others: Demonstration of anti-rejection effects of blood transfusion in kidney transplantation
1961–	K. Stern, R. Finn, V. Freda, J. Gorman, C. Clarke and others: Passive transfer of Rh antibodies prevents Rh immunization

Table 4. The era of fractionation of whole blood and plasma – the 1970s.

1955–	C. Finch, E. Simon, H. Yoshikawa, M. Nakao and others: Purines and purine nucleosides improve the storage of red cells at 4°C
1965	C. de Verdier, C. Högman, G. Bartlett and others: ACD-adenine in routine use for RBC storage
1975–	C. Högman, A. Lovric and others: Introduction of additive systems for the storage of red cells (SAG, SAGM, Circle-pack)
1950–	A. Smith, J. Lovelock, J. Farrant, H. Meryman, H. Sloviter, R. Valeri and others: Long-term storage of red cells as well as some other blood cells is applied using suitable cryoprotectants
1975	Increasing understanding that the blood components are seldom needed in the proportion they appear in the healthy blood donor
1970s	Hemapheresis methods are being used for
	– production of blood components
	– removal of non-dialysable substances from the blood, e.g. toxic agents, antibodies
1963	A. Liley: Intrauterine transfusion to the fetus in highly Rh immunized mothers
1970s	Granulocyte transfusions in patients with transient bone marrow aplasia
1944–	E. Cohn and others: Ethanol methods of plasma fractionation are taken into practical use: Albumin, fibrinogen, gammaglobulin
1958	B. & M. Blombäck and others: Factor VIII concentrates for clinical use (fraction I-O)
1965	J. Pool and others: Cryoprecipitate as a factor VIII concentrate
1975–	Increased need of plasma for fractionation to satisfy the need of albumin and factor VIII

[5], was to a great extent responsible for the progress and success, because the scarce serum reagents sufficed for extensive testing. The HLA system was mapped, in particular what is now called class I series of HLA antigens and against those corresponding genes. R. Ceppellini, F. Kissmeyer-Nielsen, R. Payne, J. van Rood, P. Terasaki, just to mention a few of those connected to transfusion medicine, gave valuable contributions to our understanding of what was found to be the major human histocompatibility system. Using short-term cell culture F. Bach and others showed the existence of another histocompatibility locus, included in the HLA class II series [6].

Transfusion medicine got deeply involved in transplantation immunology, being responsible for pretransplantation testing – both HLA typing and cross-matching – in many countries. Kidney transplantation became gradually a routine procedure and the attempt was to give the patient the best possible HLA match. Transplantation collaboration programs were established, such as Eurotransplant, Scandiatransplant etc. These were clearly important in the early stages of development but lost some of their importance when general immunosuppression became more effective.

A discovery of great theoretical and practical importance was the finding of K. Stern, R. Finn, V. Freda, J. Gorman, C. Clarke and others that passive transfer of IgG class Rh antibodies to a non-Rh immunized woman shortly after delivery prevented subsequent Rh immunization. This forms the end-point of a remarkable series of discoveries concerning hemolytic disease of the newborn (HDN).

The era of fractionation of whole blood and plasma – the 1970s (summarized in Table 4)

During liquid storage of whole blood or red cell concentrate the erythrocyte content of ATP gradually diminishes, a phenomenon related to loss of viability. The addition of purines and purine nucleosides to the anticoagulant improved the storage conditions, as shown by C. Finch, E. Simon, H. Yoshikawa, M. Nakao and others [7]. A considerable prolongation of storage – from 3 to 5 weeks – could be obtained by simply adding a small amount of adenine to the anticoagulant. Such systems were taken into practical use in Sweden from 1965 [7]. A problem that remained was that the amount of glucose, necessary for red cell metabolism, could be insufficient if the red cell units were highly concentrated by removal of the great part of plasma.

In the 1950s and 1960s whole blood transfusion strongly dominated in transfusion medicine in spite of the fact that an appropriate technique for blood component preparation – closed plastic bag system – was available. However, a gradual understanding arose that the blood components rarely are needed in the proportion they appear in the healthy blood donor. Good arguments for the superiority of blood component therapy were presented in the 1960s-1970s and became part of medical education on all levels.

The resistance among surgeons and anesthesists against the use of red cell concentrates was partly of a practical nature; the viscosity of the preparations was often so high that they could not be given rapidly without previously being diluted with saline. This was considered an obstacle in large, acute blood loss. In 1975 we showed [see 7] that red cells could be stored in a simple and pharmacologically non-controversial additive solution, containing sodium chloride, adenine, and glucose. To allow a maximum harvest of plasma mannitol was later added to the medium. A similar principle was applied by Lovric et al. The additive solution principle allowed improved standardization and quality, when the major part of leukocytes and platelets were removed, thereby reducing some of the side effects. Also a sufficient supply of nutrients – glucose and adenine – was provided to the red cells without contaminating the plasma.

Long-term storage of blood cells became available, when it was shown by A. Smith, J. Lovelock, J. Farrant, H. Meryman, H. Sloviter, R. Valeri and others that the cells could be protected from the freezing-thawing injury if mixed with a cryoprotectant and frozen under certain precautions. For red cells in transfusion volumes this means in practice sufficiently high concentrations of glycerol [see 1,p.152]. During about a decade frozen red cells were used at a few percent of total transfusions. The major indications were quality considerations; in the process of washing off the glycerol they became depleted of leukocytes. It was hoped that washing would also reduce the hepatitis risk. This latter effect seems to be minor, however. When more effective and less expensive methods for leukocyte depletion became available, the interest in frozen storage has been concentrated to cases where real long-term storage is needed, mainly rare blood types.

In the 1960s manual apheresis had been introduced for the preparation of blood components other than red cells. In addition, automated techniques were developed which allowed processing of large volumes of blood, either using continuous or discontinuous apheresis systems. Since the turnover of leukocytes, platelets, and plasma proteins are so much shorter than that of the red cells, the interval between donations could be reduced without hazard to the donor.

The new apheresis procedures have been applied during the 1970s at a large scale, both for production of blood components, as indicated above, and for treatment of patients. The latter concerns high molecular weight substances, such as some toxic agents and antibodies, which are not dialysable, and which have to be removed from the circulation.

In 1944 E. Cohn described a technique to separate plasma proteins using the following variables: Different concentrations of ethanol, ionic strength, and pH. The plasma proteins were precipitated, and could be separated by centrifugation. With or without further purification steps more or less highly purified plasma protein fractions could be obtained. Plasma fractionation institutions were established already in the late 1940s and early 1950s, producing a few fractions for clinical use, mainly albumin, fibrinogen and gammaglobulin. Albumin could be pasteurized, i.e. heat treated, and was found to have very few side effects except for overload of the circulation. Fibrinogen, on the other hand, had a very high risk of transmitting hepatitis, and was used with great restriction, therefore. Gammaglobulin preparations had to be used in intramuscular injections, causing systemic complications when used intravenously.

In the late 1950s B. and M. Blombäck showed that a factor VIII preparation could be obtained in a modified Cohn fraction from fresh or fresh-frozen plasma, the so-called fraction I-O [8]. This preparation contained also the von Willebrand factor but was not highly purified. In 1965 J. Pool described a technique to make a factor VIII concentrate in a very simple way by freezing and thawing plasma, and separating the resulting cryoprecipitate by centrifugation [9]. Also this preparation contained the von Willebrand factor. For one to two decades these two preparations implied a major change for the hemophiliacs in many countries. Effective treatment of and prophylaxis against bleeding now became a reality.

During the 1970s the demand of albumin and factor VIII preparations – and of plasma as source material – increased strongly. Furthermore, it became possible to produce a purified factor VIII preparation, however lacking the

Table 5. The need of donor blood.

- To cover the need of red cells 45–55 blood donations per 1000 inhabitants per year
- 100% blood component additive system for maximum harvest of plasma provides 15 kg plasma per 1000 inhabitants per year at 55 donations per 1000 inhabitants per year
- If 5 kg per 1000 inhabitants per year is used for transfusion purposes, including platelets, 10 kg plasma per 1000 inhabitants per year is available for fractionation
- If the fractionation yield is 200 IU factor VIII per kg plasma 2 IU factor VIII per inhabitant will be obtained
- If the use of factor VIII is >2 IU per inhabitant additional plasma has to be produced, e.g. by plasmapheresis, or recombinant factor VIII be used

---

von Willebrand factor, starting from cryoprecipitate. The major problem was that the yield was very poor, further stressing the demand of source plasma. Immunoglobulin preparations without polymers and other denaturation products allowed intravenous administration (IGIV), which has been very important when high-doses were needed for an appropriate effect. More recently, other plasma products, antithrombin III, C1-esterase inhibitor, factor VII and others have become available in addition to highly purified preparations of factor VIII and factor IX. Of great practical and economical importance has been the improved yield from the source material that has been obtained in recent years. Responsible for the supply of plasma products has been both non-profit and for-profit organizations; the latter had 63% of the international market in 1987.

In order to supply plasma for fractionation two possibilities were available: 1) to apply blood component production and restrictive use, saving plasma when this was not important to transfuse; 2) to apply apheresis technique for plasma donation, by which a larger volume of plasma can be obtained from a limited number of donors and the interval between the donations can be drastically shortened. Plasma from component production has dominated the not-for-profit sector, whereas the plasmapheresis production has dominated the for-profit sector.

An interesting question is how much plasma that is needed for self-sufficiency within a country or other geographic region. So far, this has depended mainly on two factors: 1) how much factor VIII that is used; 2) the yield of factor VIII from source plasma. As is shown in the example in Table 5 self-sufficiency can be obtained within a blood component program if: 1) not more than one third of the total available plasma is used in unfractionated form; 2) an optimal, additive system for blood component production is used, allowing a maximal harvest of plasma; 3) the yield of factor VIII from source plasma in the fractionation process is above 200 IU per kg; and 4) the use of factor VIII does not exceed 2 IU per inhabitant per year. If more factor VIII is

Table 6. The era of infectious diseases transmissible with blood products – the 1980s.

1981	A new disease – AIDS – is discovered. Its causing agent can be transmitted with blood products
1983–1984	L. Montagnier, R. Gallo and others: The Human Immunodeficiency Virus (HIV) is identified
1985–	Methods for detection of anti-HIV become available for screening
1985–	Methods for virus inactivation in plasma products are applied
1989	HCV is identified as the major cause of NANBH
1980s	Dramatic increase of the need of plasma for FVIII. Highly purified preparations cause low yield
–	New plasma products are developed: IGIV, AT-III, FVII, C1-INA a.o. special products. The indications for their respective use increase
–	Request for national self-sufficiency with plasma – 100% blood component therapy – additional plasma donation by apheresis

needed, supplementary plasmapheresis seems to be the best way, unless the needs are not satisfied by other types of preparations, such as recombinant factor VIII.

The era of infectious diseases transmissible with blood products – the 1980s (summarized in Table 6)

In 1981 a new disease, AIDS, was discovered in the USA. Suspicions early arose that this disease was caused by a virus and that it could be transmitted with contaminated blood products. In 1983-84 the virus, later called human immunodeficiency virus (HIV), had been isolated through the work of L. Montagnier and R. Gallo and their respective co-workers, and a method to detect antibodies against the virus was developed. Somewhat surprisingly it was found that persons with circulating HIV antibodies almost always also carry the virus. Thus no protecting immunity occurred, as was the case in most other infectious diseases. In 1985 methods suitable for mass screening of blood donors were available and became widely applied.

The fact that infectious diseases could be transmitted with blood was well known since the 1940s. Concern had been shown for the risk of transmitting bacterial infections such as syphilis and parasitical diseases such as malaria, even if these quantitatively represented a minor problem. Hepatitis was the greatest threat. Screening for hepatitis B was instituted in the late 1960s and made hepatitis B a largely preventible disease. However, there existed other transmissible virus or viruses causing the so-called non-A,non-B hepatitis (NANBH). The recent discovery of hepatitis C virus, HCV, promises to be the major NANBH virus and selection of anti-HCV negative donors a further important step toward safer transfusion, hopefully making posttransfusion hepatitis a rare event.

Table 7. Number of patients contracting HIV infection via blood products in Sweden 1980–1990.

	80	81	82	83	84	85	86	87	88	89	90
Blood components*	6	3	14	20	30	12	0	0	0	0	0
Plasma fractions**	21	36	15	11	1	2	1	0	0	0	0

* Eight more cases are recorded where the year of infection is unknown.

** Six more cases are recorded where the year of infection is unknown. All except four cases were caused by factor VIII concentrates prepared from non-Swedish plasma. Four hemophilia B persons contacted the infection via one batch of infected factor IX concentrate prepared from Swedish plasma.

Before 1980 the people working in transfusion services seem to have been more concerned about the risks of transfusion than those treating patients. This attitude has now been dramatically changed. The pendulum has tended to swing to the other extreme: An enormous and often overexagerated fear among patients (as well as health care workers) for contracting HIV or other infections from blood products. Although the risk of transmitting HIV this way should not be neglected – it clearly is a reality in certain areas – the measures taken in to-day's transfusion medicine make the risk an extremely small one in most Western countries. This may be illustrated by the development in Sweden during the 1980s (Table 7). A frightening development was retrospectively seen in the early 1980s. The good, computerized registration systems in transfusion medicine made the look-back studies very effective. The hemophiliacs became infected mostly in the early 1980s and – with respect to factor VIII – only through products made from non-Swedish donors. This trend was aborted in 1985, when anti-HIV testing started. From 1986 and on no transfusion transmitted HIV infection has been observed, representing products from 2 million blood collections.

An important spin-off effect of this risk awareness is the development of several effective virus reducing methods for treating plasma products. This has given the result that not only albumin solutions but also coagulation factor preparations and other fractionated products can be considered safe with respect to all presently known viruses that can be transmitted with blood. Methods now become available for anti-viral treatment of plasma. If it will be possible also to treat blood cells is still an open question.

The 1980s – Also the era of changing transfusion patterns (summarized in Table 8)

Another trend in the 1980s has been the changing pattern of blood product consumption. The use of red cells has decreased slightly in most countries. The rising use of granulocyte concentrate in the 1970s has turned into very

Table 8. The 1980s – Also the era of changing transfusion patterns.

The consumption pattern for blood components changes:
− use of red cells decreases slightly
− use of platelets increases dramatically
− use of granulocytes decreases

Therapeutic refractoriness in platelet-dependent patients causes problems:
− need of and supply with platelets from HLA compatible donors
− platelet cross-match testing an alternative

Technical development:
− improved methods for hemapheresis
− automation of blood component production
− highly effective filters for leukocyte removal reduce the occurrence of HLA immunization
− reduction of lymphocyte immunogenicity by UV irradiation

Recombinant human factor VIII is produced, tested in hemophilia patients, and found effective

Hormones which govern the formation and maturation of blood cells and regulate the immune system are identified and produced:
− interferons (first produced from donor leukocytes, later by recombinant technique)
− erythropoietin – reduce transfusions in patients with nephrologically dependent bone marrow depression (useful in pre-operative blood deposit)
− interleukins and colony stimulating factors

Interleukins, growth factors etc. are being used:
− for treatment of patients
− for treatment of isolated cell fractions, e.g. obtained by apheresis

---

limited use in the 1980s. Instead the demand of platelets has increased tremendously in the treatment of the iatrogenic, transient bone marrow aplasia, which follows modern aggressive treatment of hematological malignancies and bone marrow transplantation. Here, therapeutic refractoriness to platelet transfusion has been a problem, mainly the result of repeated transfusion of leukocyte contaminated blood components. In order to achieve compatibility, platelets have been produced by apheresis of HLA compatible donors. Platelet cross-matching procedures have also proven their value.

At the end of the 1980s very effective filtration techniques have become available for real leukocyte depletion of red cell and platelet preparations. Again the consumption pattern seems to be changing. Highly leukocyte depleted platelet concentrates do not immunize the recipient, at least to the same extent as the leukocyte contaminated products did. Using leukocyte depleted products the demand for HLA compatible products has decreased most considerably. Another opportunity which shows great promises is to change the immunizing power of the lymphocytes by irradiation with ultraviolet light. The technique may be useful as an alternative to filter depletion or as a means of inducing tolerogenic effects.

The fear for transfusion transmitted infection has stimulated the interest in autologous transfusion, both cell saving procedures in conjunction with surgery, and predeposit of autologous blood components some time before an operation. It has been shown that a considerable percentage of all patients demanding transfusion, 25% in a study in Milan [see 10], can be sufficiently supplied with autologous blood alone. In order to speed up regeneration of red cells human recombinant erythropoietin can be of benefit [see 10].

Blood component production traditionally has been labour intensive, completely manual, and not very well standardized. In Europe three new methods of automating component production have been developed, all of them invented in blood banks, and all of them in large-scale practical use. This has resulted in much better standardization of the products.

In addition an important development of the apheresis techniques has occurred, making the machines safer and easier to manage. In several countries they have been used at a large-scale for the supply of plasma and platelets. But also fascinating new applications have been developed which imply harvesting of leukocytes and stem cells from the peripheral blood, used to supplement or replace bone marrow stem cells in transplantation, or for gene repair in hereditary diseases such as adenosine deaminase deficiency (ADA).

A number of hormones with regularly functions in the hematopoietic and immune systems have become available, first produced by stimulation of donor leukocytes (interferons) or platelets (platelet derived growth factor), later produced by recombinant DNA technology. These hormones are now used in the direct treatment of patients, such as erythropoietin in uremia-induced anemia, but also for treating cells obtained from patients by apheresis and, after manipulation, re-injected in the patient to obtain certain effects. Examples of such hormones are interleukins (IL) and colony stimulating growth factors (e.g. G-CSF and GM-CSF).

Transfusion medicine in the 1990s (summarized in Table 9)

It has been claimed that blood products derived from human donors is obsolete and that they will soon be replaced by industrially made pharmaceuticals. In the view of the author this is not likely to occur during this side of the year 2000 and not during the first decade of the new century either.

There is no real substitute for red cells in sight. Polymerized hemoglobin solutions, which seem to be a realistic possibility as combined blood volume expanders and oxygen carriers in moderate blood loss – when long-term effects are not necessary – have moved very slowly and are still not available for large scale clinical trials. Thus red cells will be needed, although probably smaller extent than now. Plasma as obtained in blood component production will be the likely source for many products, simply for economical reasons.

Table 9. Transfusion medicine in the 1990s.

No real substitute for red cells in sight:
- polymerized hemoglobin solution may act as a combined volume expander and oxygen carrier when long-term effects are not necessary

Increased emphasis on safety and efficacy:
- extended use of autologous transfusion:
  - blood saving procedures
  - predeposit, with or without EPO, in elective surgery
- improved selection of safe donors

Blood components, cellular products:
- improved additive solutions for red cells and platelets
- possibly: virus reducing procedures

Blood component plasma:
- fractionated into plasma products
- virus reduction in unfractionated plasma

Trace proteins, e.g. factor VIII, partly plasma derived, partly recombinant

Increased use of hemapheresis in patients:
- to harvest stem cells and/or lymphocytes:
  - for transplantation
  - for in vitro manipulation – "gene repair"

Development of the antigen chemistry of blood and tissue cells and of the mechanisms for manipulation of immune response, eventually allowing xeno-transplantation

---

Trace proteins like factor VIII are likely to be produced by recombinant technology, replacing plasma factor VIII to the extent this is made by apheresis to prepare factor VIII only. However, IGIV is now increasing rapidly in use in spite of its large expense. Considering the complexity and multispecificity of the immunoglobulins it seems likely that they will be produced from plasma, at least for several of the present therapeutic indications.

The use of predeposit procedures is likely to increase. What is needed is greater interest from the transfusion medicine people to set up the organization for it and to give the appropriate information to patients and medical staff.

The demand of safety will probably continue to increase, requiring improved procedures for donor selection. This means that the cost will go further up. The question arises whether it will be possible to get rid of some regulations which have become clearly obsolete and of no value; an example may be the requirement of a negative syphilis antibody test concerning plasma for fractionation. Even if the plasma would contain syphilis spirochaetes, which is extremely unlikely, the transfer of living organisms through the alcohol fractionation procedure to the final products is impossible.

A major issue is how to manipulate the immune system of a transplant recipient in such a way that general immune suppression will be unnecessary, in other words to obtain specific tolerance. It seems likely that these problems eventually will be solved, allowing improved allotransplantation and possibly also xeno-transplantation. The tasks involved in such activities would seem natural for those transfusion medicine people already deeply involved in the laboratory service, preparatively and/or diagnostically, to organ and bone marrow transplantation.

References

1. Mollison PL, Engelfriet CP, Contreras M. Blood transfusion in clinical medicine. Blackwell Scientific Publications, 8th ed., Oxford 1987.
2. Mollison PL. Blood transfusion in clinical medicine. Blackwell Scientific Publications, 5th ed., Oxford 1972.
3. Diamond LK. Erythroblastosis foetalis or haemolytic disease of the newborn. Proc Roy Soc Med 1947;40:546.
4. Allen FH jr, Diamond LK, Vaughan VCIII. Erythroblastosis fetalis. VI. Prevention of kernicterus. Amer J Dis Child 1950;80:779.
5. Terasaki PI, McClelland JC, Park MS, McCurdy B. Microdroplet lymphocyte cytoxicity test, in: Manual of tissue typing techniques. DHEW publ (NIH) 74-545. Government Printing Office, Washington DC.
6. Bach FH, Voynow NK. One-way stimulation in mixed lymphocyte cultures. Science 1966;153:545.
7. Högman CF (ed). Liquid storage of human erythrocytes, in: Blood separation and plasma fractionation. New York: Wiley-Liss 1991:63-97.
8. Blombäck M. Purification of antihemophilic globulin. I. Some studies on the stability of the antihemophilic globulin activity in fraction I-O and a method for its partial separation from fibrinogen. Ark Kemi 1958;12:387-96.
9. Pool JG, Shannon AE. Production of high potency concentrates of antihemophilic globulin in a closed bag system. N Engl J Med 1965;273:1443-7.
10. Högman CF. Blood transfusion, blood products and autologous transfusion. Current opinion in Anaesthesiology 1991;4:218-23.

TRANSFUSION MEDICINE: THE IMPACT OF BIOTECH-NOLOGY, GROWTH FACTORS, AND BIOENGINEERING

H.G. Klein

Introduction

Basic science advances coupled with sophisticated new instrumentation have been moving the discipline of Transfusion Medicine beyond its traditional role as supplier of blood components into such evolving fields as cancer cellular biotherapy, bone marrow transplantation, and gene therapy. Bioreactor culture systems, improved techniques of cell separation, and applied molecular biology are a few of the areas that promise to revolutionize transfusion practices [1]. However few discoveries have made the immediate impact or captured the imagination to the extent that have a series of regulatory molecules known as cytokines, interleukins, or hematopoietic growth factors.

Investigation and application of growth factor biology promise to change the face of Transfusion Medicine by the millennium.

Hematopoietic cytokines

Through recombinant DNA technology, more than a dozen interleukins, erythropoietin, and several myeloid growth factors have been identified, characterized and produced in volumes suitable for pharmaceutical purposes. The first growth factor licensed for human use, recombinant human erythropoietin (rhEPO), a lineage-specific glycoprotein capable of stimulating the bone marrow to produce red cells, has already influenced transfusion services dramatically. In a study of 330 patients with chronic renal disease, researchers using rhEPO almost eliminated transfusions, compared with 0.52 units per patient per month transfused during the six months proceeding therapy. If these data can be extrapolated to the estimated 25,000 Americans with transfusion-dependent end-stage renal disease, the national savings in red cells may approach 500,000 units annually [2]. More recently, evidence indicates that rhEPO can reduce the transfusion requirements of selected patients with AIDS and cancer, and possibly of patients undergoing cardiac surgery. The drug has already been approved for the former two indications [3,4,5]. Of special interest to transfusion services is the reported increase in autologous blood that can be collected and stored, if rhEPO is added to the prospective patient's phlebotomy regimen [6]. While this application of rhEPO is expensive and still of unproved practical value, its real importance lies in the principle of using recombinant human growth factors to improve the availability of blood components.

Blood banks are also beginning to feel the impact of recombinant myeloid growth factors. One of the early hopes of the designers of blood cell separators was that these instruments could be used to collect sufficient numbers of granulocytes to support leukopenic patients with bacterial and fungal infections. The current instruments can harvest 2 to 4×10^{10} granulocytes if the donor is stimulated with an adrenocorticosteroid and if a starch or gelatin solution is used to enhance buffy coat separation in the collection process. The difficulty in collecting and storing large numbers of granulocytes, the potential side effects, and perhaps a new generation of antibiotics has limited the use of granulocyte transfusions. However mortality for severely neutropenic patients with documented infections remains at about ten percent [7]. The two major myeloid growth factors, granulocyte colony-stimulating factor (G-CSF) and granulocyte-macrophage colony-stimulating factor (GM-CSF) have already been used to shorten the severe neutropenia that accompanies cancer chemotherapy and bone marrow transplantation [8,9]. More speculative, perhaps, is the potential use of these cytokines to stimulate volunteer donors, especially those of a desired HLA type, to provide large numbers of granulocytes and mononuclear cells for transfusion purposes. The toxicity of both growth factors appears to be dose related. At low doses, both are capable of evoking a substantial leukocytosis with minimal adverse effects. Furthermore, both laboratory studies and in vivo evidence indicate that exposure to GM-CSF may enhance several granulocyte functions and prolong granulocyte survival [10-12]. These observations suggest the possibility of developing a leukocyte transfusion component containing large numbers of "super cells".

Management of disseminated fungal infections is a growing problem in granulocytopenic patients, especially in those with repeated or prolonged episodes of granulocytopenia. One approach that we have taken in collaboration with the pediatric oncology branch of the National Cancer Institute is to collect, purify, and activate circulating human monocytes. While monocytes constitute only about five percent of circulating leukocytes, techniques combining standard blood cell separators and counterflow centrifugal elutriation can produce preparations with more than 10^9 leukocytes of which 90% or more are monocytes. Monocytes secrete a variety of cytokines including interleukin-1 and tumour necrosis factor (TNF) and play multiple roles in host defense including antigen presentation in the immune response and phagocytosis. In addition, cytokine-activated monocytes have anti-fungal activity, at least *in vitro* [13]. Unlike granulocyte collections monocyte concentrates can be stored at 4°C and cryopreserved in dimethylsulfoxide. A single study with homologous monocytes labelled with Indium-111 in our laboratory and activated with GM-CSF, demonstrated cell migration to the site of tissue invasion by aspergillus. These limited data suggest to us that monocyte transfusion is an area of investigation worth further study.

Another area related to transfusion and amenable to application of hemato-poietic growth factors involve the expansion, harvest, manipulation, storage, and reinfusion of autologous bone marrow progenitor cells. Such cells can be prepared from standard bone marrow aspirations, but progenitors also circu-late in small numbers in the peripheral blood of normal subjects. GM-CSF has been shown to expand both bone marrow and circulating human hematopoietic progenitor compartments [14-16]. Some Transfusion Medicine Departments already process bone marrow and harvest peripheral blood progenitor cells for autologous marrow reconstitution of patients treated with aggressive che-motherapy. The initial studies indicate that circulating progenitors mobilized with GM-CSF, alone or combined with autologous marrow re-infusion, can accelerate marrow recovery in patients who receive myeloablative therapy [17,18]. Preliminary studies suggest further that G-CSF and interleukin-3 (IL-3), a growth factor that acts on earlier progenitors, also expand the pool of circulating progenitors. Combinations of growth factors act synergistically in promoting hematopoiesis in primates.

These therapies are still investigational; they suffer from primitive "stem cell" assay techniques, limited methods of early progenitor enrichment, and lack of standards for collection, storage, and preparation of the infusion com-ponent. Nevertheless, this is clearly an area of future involvement for Trans-fusion Medicine.

Cellular biotherapy

The ability to collect, expand, and activate mononuclear cells ex vivo has op-ened another area in which transfusion specialists should play an important future role, the adoptive immunotherapy of malignant disease. Several differ-ent cell types have been proposed and used experimentally as candidate agents for adoptive immunotherapy. Autologous natural killer (NK) cells or a species of NK, the lymphokine-activated killer (LAK) cell, tumour infiltrating lym-phocytes (TIL), and monocytes have all been collected, expanded, activated, and infused into patients with different, widely metastatic malignancies [18].

In the few clinical studies with interferon-activated monocytes, another use of a lymphokine, cells were infused intraperitoneally in patients with pelvic carcinomatosis. Radiolabelled cell trafficking studies and "second-look" lapa-rotomies both proved encouraging, and adverse effects of treatment were few and mild. There has been little done to follow up the preliminary studies des-pite the early enthusiasm for this treatment [19].

In contrast, an enormous amount of basic laboratory study, animal ex-perimentation, and clinical information has accumulated with lymphocytes activated with the lymphokine, interleukin-2 (IL-2). The initial clinical studies of these cells collected with cell separators from patients with a variety of ma-lignancies, expanded in culture for four days, and reinfused together with high doses of IL-2, showed a 13 to 25% patient response rate, but more importantly, demonstrated long-term disease-free survival in several patients. Certain tumours, especially renal cell carcinoma, melanoma, and lymphoma appear to be the best candidates for future clinical study. This therapy has major toxic effects, but these seem to be related primarily to the high doses of IL-2 employed, rather than to the cells.

Harvesting lymphocytes from resected melanoma and expanding them in long-term culture with IL-2 produce TIL, cells that seem more specific and potent than LAK cells. These cells traffic to tumour sites, expand under the influence of IL-2, and can be cryopreserved. Clinical studies indicate that TIL are effective in patients with melanoma and may persist for months in the circulation and at metastatic sites [20,21]. From a transfusion medicine standpoint, harvest, preparation, storage, quality control, labelling and cryopreservation lie within our area of expertise, and we should plan to participate fully as these therapies move from the research laboratory to the bedside.

Somatic cell gene therapy

Using many of the same techniques involved in adoptive immunotherapy, researchers at the National Institutes of Health recently performed the first therapeutic human somatic cell gene insertion, effectively correcting the rare inherited disorder, adenosine deaminase (ADA) deficiency, in two children. The team selected the T-lymphocyte as a vehicle for gene transfer for several reasons: 1) the T-lymphocyte is a target cell in ADA deficiency; 2) lymphocytes are readily available as a single cell suspension, easy to culture or cryopreserve, and readily transfused; 3) although lymphocytes are not pluripotential stem cells, they are long-lived and can be expanded in vivo by immunization; 4) long-term cultures offers potential advantages of multiple gene insertions, selection of expressing cells, and opportunity to perform safety testing. In this protocol, leukocytes were harvested by cytapheresis, separated with a density gradient, and placed into wells of culture plates for gene insertion. The cells were stimulated to devide with a combination of monoclonal anti-CD3 and IL-2, and transduced with a genetically engineered incomplete retroviral vector containing the ADA gene. The dividing cells were expanded in plastic blood bags and eventually reinfused to the patients. Preliminary data indicated that the gene-corrected cells are surviving for months, expressing ADA, and correcting the immunologic and clinical defects in both children.

The first gene-modified cells transfused to cancer patients were used for diagnostic purposes [21]. However the ability to modify these cells, for example by inserting additional TNF genes or genes that otherwise modify the lymphocyte, raises almost limitless possibilities for cellular therapy of cancer.

Eventually, somatic cell gene therapy may well involve the hematopoietic stem cell. Preliminary studies have been frustrated by the difficulties of isolating the earliest progenitor, inserting genes into a quiescent cell, and effecting stable gene expression during subsequent cellular differentiation. The availability of an array of growth factors, including the recently cloned stem cell factor *c-kit* ligand (KL), lends an air of optimism to research in this area [22].

Scientists are still a long way from growing blood for transfusion in the laboratory. However advances in basic science and biotechnology make the prospect more than science fiction. After all, few physicians believed that gene therapy would open this decade and few blood centres believed that this technology would flourish in their laboratories. Translating these exciting discoveries from the research laboratory to the bedside will require personnel experienced in harvesting cells from patients, facilities for manipulating and storing or cryopreserving the components in a safe and sterile fashion, standards for labelling, quality assurance, and issue, and experience in infusion therapy. Scientists, physicians, and technologists, trained in the Transfusion Medicine of the future should play an integral role in these therapies.

References

1. Chernoff AI, Klein HG, Sherman LA (eds). Research opportunities in Transfusion Medicine. Transfusion 1989;29:711-42.
2. Eschbach JW, Abdulhabi MH, Browne JK, et al. Recombinant human erythropoietin in anemic patients with end-stage renal disease. Ann Intern Med 1989;111: 992-1000.
3. Fischl M, Galpin JE, Levine JD, et al. Recombinant human erythropoietin for patients with AIDS treated with Zidovudine. N Engl J Med 1990;322:1488-93.
4. Miller CB, Jones RJ, Piandosi S, Abeloff, Spivak JL. Decreased erythropoietin response in patients with the anemia of cancer. N Engl J Med 1990;322:1689-92.
5. Watanabe Y, Fuse K, Konishi T,et al. Autologous blood transfusion with recombinant human erythropoietin in heart operation. Ann Thorac Surg 1991;51:767-72.
6. Goodnough LT, Rudnick S, Stehling LC, et al. Predeposited autologous blood for elective surgery: A national multicenter study. N Engl J Med 1989;321:1163-68.
7. Pizzo PA, Hathorn JW, Hiemenz J, et al. A randomized trial comparing ceftazidime alone with combination antibiotic therapy in cancer patients with fever and neutropenia. N Engl J Med 1986;315:552-8.
8. Crawford J, Ozer H, Stoller R, et al. Reduction by granulocyte colony stimulating factor of fever and neutropenia induced by chemotherapy in patients with small-cell lung cancer. N Engl J Med 1991;325:164-70.
9. Nemunaitis J, Rabinowe SN, Singer JW, et al. Recombinant granulocyte-macrophage colony stimulating factor after autologous bone marrow transplantation with lymphoid cancer. N Engl J Med 1991;324:1773-78.
10. Weisbart RH, Kwan L, Golde DW, Gasson JC. Human GM-CSF primes neutrophils for enhanced oxidative metabolism in response to the major physiological chemoattractants. Blood 1987;69:18-21.
11. Sullivan R, Fredette JP, Socinski M, et al. Enhancement of superoxide release by granulocytes harvested from patients receiving granulocyte-macrophage colony-stimulating factor. Brit J Haematol 1989;71:475-89.
12. Begley CG, Lopez AF, Nicola NA, et al. Purified colony-stimulating factors enhance the survival of human neutrophils and eosinophils *in vitro*: A rapid and sensitive microassay for colony-stimulating factors. Blood 1986;68:162-66.

158

13. Smith PD, Lamerson CL, Banks SM, et al. Granulocyte-macrophage colony-stimulating factor augments human monocyte fungicidal activity for *Candida albicans*. J Inf Dis 1990;161:999-1005.
14. Aglietta M, Piacibello W, Sanavio F, et al. Kinetics of human hemopoietic cells after *in vivo* administration of granulocyte-macrophage colony stimulating factor. J Clin Invest 1988;83:551-57.
15. Siena S, Bregni M, Brando B, Ravagnani F, Bonadonna G, Gianni AM. Circulation of CD34$^+$ hematopoietic stem cells in the peripheral blood of high-dose cyclophosphamide-treated patients: Enhancement by intravenous recombinant human granulocyte-macrophage colony-stimulating factor. Blood 1989;74:1905-14.
16. Haas R, Ho AD, Bredthauer U, et al. Successful autologous transplantation of blood stem cells mobilized with recombinant human granulocyte-macrophage colony-stimulating factor. Exp Hematol 1990:1894-98.
17. Gianni AM, Bregni M, Siena S, et al. Recombinant human granulocyte-macrophage colony-stimulating factor reduces hematologic toxicity and widens clinical applicability of high-dose cyclophosphamide treatment in breast cancer and non-Hodgkins lymphoma. J Clin Oncol 1990;8:768-78.
18. Klein HG, Leitman SF. Adoptive immunotherapy in the treatment of malignant disease. Transfusion 1989;29:170-78.
19. Stevenson HC, Foon KA, Sugarbaker PH. Ex vivo activation of killer monocytes and their application to the treatment of human cancer. J Clin Apheresis 1988;4:114-21.
20. Topalian S, Solomon D, Avis FP, et al. Immunotherapy of patients with advanced cancer using tumor-infiltrating lymphocytes and recombinant interleukin-2: A pilot study. J Clin Oncol 1988;6:839-53.
21. Rosenberg SA, Aebersold P, Cornetta K, et al. Gene transfer into humans – immunotherapy of patients with advanced melanoma, using tumor-infiltrating lymphocytes modified by retroviral gene transduction. N Engl J Med 1990;323:570-78.
22. Anderson DM, Lyman SD, Baird A, et al. Molecular cloning of mast cell growth factor, a hematopoietin that is active in both membrane and soluble forms. Cell 1990;63:235.

THE SANGUIS PROJECT

H.J. ten Duis, D.B.L. McClelland, A.M. Giovanetti on behalf of the study group[1]

Blood is a human tissue and in biological terms, the administration of blood has more in common with the transplantation of bone marrow or a solid organ than with the administration of a pharmacological agent such as an antibiotic. The biological risks associated with transfusion are well known and, of course, it also carries substantial financial costs.

The decisions associated with undertaking a tissue or organ transplantation are recognized as being complex, high level clinical decisions which require the analysis of extensive information about both patient and donor. Furthermore, the rules which govern successful transplantation have been derived over many years of disciplined scientific and clinical experiments which have defined with increasing precision the clinical situations in which, first of all, the benefits to the patient outweigh the risks, and, second, the costs of the procedure are justified by the value of measurable outcomes showing benefit to the patient like quality assured life years and a decreased morbidity. These decisions are taken by clinical staff with a high level of expertise in very specialized areas including hematology and transplant immunology.

While it is true that some transfusion decisions are taken with similar attention, it is well known that in a high proportion of cases, blood is seen simply as a useful red fluid to be ordered without profound thought, often by junior doctors and inexperienced staff. It is not seldom given in arbitrary quantities to achieve undefined clinical or physiological end points, like, for example, to improve the colour of the patient.

The improvement of clinical transfusion practice therefore requires:
– a greatly improved basis of data to help establish, with precision, the indications for transfusion in a given patient or patient group; and
– a major effort to increase the awareness of clinicians about the need to examine and audit present practice to identify major variations in transfusion policy and ensure that practice is brought into line with standards which reflect the best information we have available at present.

1. See Table 1.

The SANGUIS project addressed the second of these points. It arose out of studies carried out in Milan by Dr. Giovanetti and her colleagues which showed that in their hospitals there was a substantial over-use of blood transfusion resources. For example, much of the blood which was ordered, was not transfused, one third of patients were given red cell transfusions showing a postoperative hematocrit greater than 36% and in 75% of operations, fresh frozen plasma was transfused as well as red cells. The few other studies available in Europe suggested that in other centres also the use of blood and blood components in surgery is less than optimal. Similar results have been published in the US and other countries.

The general hypothesis which was formed by the Milan group was that:
- substantial amounts of blood components probably were being given to patients who did not need them;
- that this carried substantial avoidable costs to the health system;
- that many patients were being needlessly exposed to transfusion hazards such as hepatitis.

It was evident, however, that there was no comprehensive body of data describing and comparing transfusion practices in Europe and in 1989 the SANGUIS[1] project was initiated to begin to collect this information.

A collaborative multidisciplinary study group, representing ten countries and four specialties, was set up to plan and carry out the study which has been led by Professor G. Sirchia and financially supported in part by the Health Service's Research Program of the CEC (Table 1).

Table 1. SANGUIS Study Group; project leader G. Sirchia, Italy.

Participants

For transfusion medicine	*For surgery*
A.M. Giovanetti, Italy	H.J. ten Duis, Netherlands
J. Jorgensen, Denmark	K. Messmer, Germany
D.B.L. McClelland, UK	
A. Maniatis, Greece	
For anesthetics and intensive care	*For comac - HSR*
P. Baele, Belgium	A. Sissouras, Greece
R.B. Carrington da Costa, Portugal	
N. Drouet, France	
A. Net Castel, Spain	

1.   SANGUIS = Safe and good use of blood in surgery.

The principle objective of the study is to assess how much, when and why blood, blood components, blood derivatives and artificial colloids are requested and transfused in specified elective surgical procedures, performed in teaching hospitals located in ten countries of the European Community. The study focuses on surgical transfusion practice because 60-80% of blood components are used in this situation and it was felt that there was already evidence to suggest the need for a more comprehensive review of practice in this area.

Six classes of surgical procedures were selected for study on the basis that they are commonly carried out, that blood is frequently ordered or used and that as far as possible the procedures could be classified within a simple protocol for data collection. The following classes of procedures were chosen:
- Cholecystectomy (chole)
- Colectomy (cole)
- Transurethral prostate resection (pr)
- First-time coronary artery bypass graft (cabg)
- Abdominal aortic aneurysmectomy (aaa)
- Total hip replacement (thr)

In most of these procedures it could also be expected that there were significant opportunities for the use of autologous transfusion like predeposit and the intraoperative salvage of shed blood.

Participating centres were large teaching hospitals selected on the basis of expressed interest in the study and willingness by appropriate staff to facilitate in the data collection exercise. This was not a rigorously selected random sample of clinical centres, and centres chosen would be expected to represent better than average standards of practice.

For each procedure 60-120 patients are to be enroled in each study centre, distributed uniformly over a one-year data collection period which finished at the end of September 1991. Centres performing large numbers of procedures enroll the first 5-10 patients arising each month in each relevant category.

Patients are enroled to the study at the time of surgery and data are collected only at or shortly after the time of discharge and are obtained only from standard clinical records. Efforts have been made to avoid influencing the quality of existing clinical practice or the recording of transfusion and no preliminary data from the study have been fed back to any of the clinical units. Thus for the study in its first phase, attempts have been made to observe existing practice without influencing it. This is one of the first presentations of the data and comes virtually at the end of the one-year database period of data collection.

The data were collected by standard protocol form and transferred to a specially developed database to allow transmission to the co-ordinating centre in Milan in Italy for analysis.

The study is assembling detailed descriptive data about the blood and blood products transfused, together with a limited set of clinical and demographic information which may provide some initial insight into the observed differences in transfusion (Table 2).

Table 2. Protocol data (in the surgical unit).

- Age, sex
- Hospital stay
- Diagnosis
- Drugs
- Anesthesia
- Blood loss
- Duration of surgery
- Blood request
- Minimum daily HCT values
- Transfusion of blood, blood components (both auto- and homologous) and derivatives, artificial colloids (nr, type, time)
- Stated reason for transfusion
- Complications of surgery, blood transfusion, autotransfusion

---

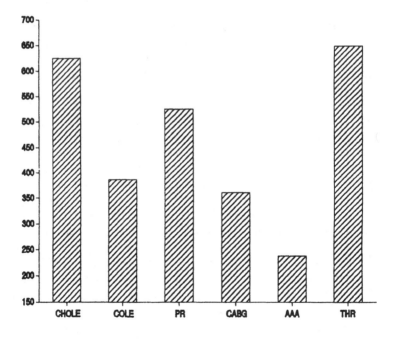

Figure 1. Patients by surgical procedure (2785).

Table 3. THR: Blood transfusion data.

	Patients			Blood units, Nr.	
	No	(% Po)	all	median	(Q1-Q3)
Transfused	550	(84.8)	2021	3	(2-4)
− autologous	76	(11.7)	217	3	(2-3)
− auto- and homologous	62	(9.5)	171 + 162	5	(3-6)
− homologous	412	(63.5)	1443	3	(2-4)
Not transfused	99	(15.2)	–	–	–

It also focuses on the quality of transfusion records by 1) looking for evidence of a written clinical order and/or transfusion explaining why a product was given, and 2) comparing transfusion data from the clinical records with matching data collected from the blood bank records.

In Figure 1 an overview of the number of patients collected in each surgical procedure is given.

To illustrate the kind of information arising from the study some interim results on a single procedure (total hip replacement) are presented, which have been drawn from data representing one third of the projected total number of patients from seven countries and 20 hospitals, of which 18 have enroled at least 20 patients. A total of 649 patient records are included in this study.

Almost universally, blood is requested for total hip replacement patients. For only 2.6% of patients no blood was requested and 0.2% were covered by a type and screen request only. The remainder had some form of crossmatch procedure reflecting a high expectation that transfusion would be needed.

85% (550/649) of patients received transfusion of blood or a component (autologous and homologous) (Table 3)

73% were exposed to one or more units of homologous donor blood. However there was great variation between clinical units. In one hospital only 44% of patients were transfused while in seven out of 20 hospitals 100% of patients received blood components.

In Figure 2 the percentage of patients in each hospitals who received red cell transfusion is shown, illustrating further the wide variation between centres.

The great majority (95%) of all components transfused, were red cells. However, in three centres a significant proportion (up to 60%) of patients received plasma transfusions. The need for any human colloid in this group of patients may be questioned.

164

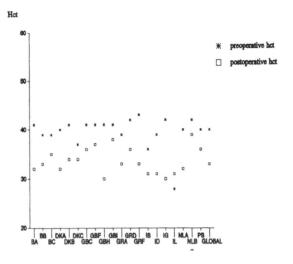

Legenda
BA, BB, BC; Belgian hospitals
DKA, DKB, DKC: Danish hospitals
GBC, GBF, GBH, GBI: British hospitals
GRA, GRD, GRF: Greek hospitals
IB, ID, IG, IL: Italian hospitals
NLA, NLB: Dutch hospitals
PB: Portugees hospital

Figure 2. THR: Blood component by hospital.

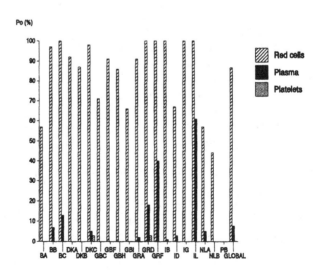

Figure 3. THR: Pre- and postoperative hematocrit.

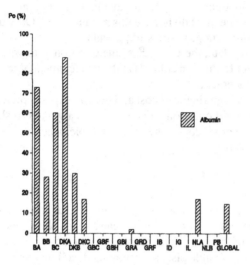

Figure 4. THR: Blood derivatives by hospital.

Looking at Table 3 in more detail, we can see the following points:
1. Only 15% of patients were managed without any transfusion;
2. 11.7% received only autologous blood, thus avoiding any exposure to homologous blood;
3. 64% received only homologous donor blood and were exposed to a median of three donors;
4. A small group of patients received both homologous and autologous blood. It is interesting to note that in this 10% of patients, a median five units was transfused.

Autologous transfusion was restricted in essence to three hospitals in Italy and two in Greece. Data from these hospitals show that it is possible to manage more than 60% of total hip replacement patients exclusively with autologous transfusion. This observation is entirely in line with a number of published studies and raises important questions about future transfusion policy for such patients and the need for relevant outcome studies to evaluate the impact of autologous transfusion programs in this group.

Pre-operative hematocrit values were remarkably uniform with the possible exception of one centre, probably associated with the more intensive use of predeposit autotransfusion (Figure 3).

Post-operative hematocrit values are less complete, but show that overall, the hematocrit falls by 17.5% despite a median of three units being transfused. It seems likely also that there may be significant differences between centres in the "accepted" level of postoperative hemoglobin which may open the way to studies relating this value to clinical outcome.

The use of human albumin is concentrated in a small number of the study centres (Figure 4) while most do not use this product at all. Only three centres use plasma in a significant proportion of patients.

These preliminary data, therefore, raise the question as to whether there is any need whatsoever for human colloids in the management of patients undergoing total hip replacement.

Albumin carries a high financial cost and plasma exposes patients to infection hazards. We should question whether there is any data to show that the use of either of these products gives any measurable benefit to the patients to justify the risks and costs.

Conclusions

Despite the fact that so far we have only begun to examine a part of the data from the SANGUIS project, we believe we can already show that it is possible to perform a study of this type in the European situation and to generate data which will stimulate valuable discussion among the clinicians responsible for surgical blood use.

Immediate future plans include:
1. To continue the quality improvement cycle by feeding back the study data to the participating units;
2. To then undertake a further period of observation to evaluate changes in practice following this first phase of the study;
3. Extend the experience, the network of contacts, and the computer software which has been developed through this study into a more widely applied audit of surgical transfusion in Europe, hopefully including participation of non-CEC European countries.

SAFETY OF TRANSFUSIONS AS WE MOVE TOWARD 2000

T.F. Zuck

"Speaking about the future is always easy because no one can contradict you. They can only have a different opinion." Stagnaro, 1989

The safety and efficacy of transfusion therapy have increased remarkably in the last decade, especially with regard to the transmission of viral diseases. Much of this progress has been driven by fears created by the emergence of the acquired immune deficiency syndrome (AIDS). As the public became aware of transfusion-transmitted AIDS, it also became concerned about other transfusion risks, most notably acquiring hepatitis. The expectations of the public concerning the safety of transfusions have grown increasingly unrealistic – it seemingly is unwilling to accept that striving for a zero-risk blood supply is futile [1].

Improvements in transfusion safety made during the past decade paradoxically pose difficulties in designing further advances in the safety systems. They may have reached the practical limits of their efficacy. Current estimates of HIV-1 transmission per unit transfused in the United States range from a low of 1 in 153,000 based on national data [2] to a high of 1 in 61,171 in a metropolitan area with high numbers of AIDS cases [3]. Thus, were the sensitivity of the enzyme-linked immunoassay (EIA) kits for antibodies to the AIDS virus, HIV-1, substantially improved, any increase in transfusion safety would be trivial and unlikely to be measurable.

Similarly, studies of improvements in donor screening procedures recently advocated suggest that, although donor comprehension will improve, only marginal increases in donor self-deferral will be achieved [4].

Because fine-tuning existing screening and safety measures is unlikely to impart significant additional safety, in the future alternative strategies to improve the safety of the blood supply will be explored by blood centres and clinical services.

In this essay, three of these strategies will be discussed:
- developing additional ways to avoid homologous transfusions;
- using quality and process engineering to reduce blood centre production and distribution errors; and
- pursuing methods to inactivate blood components.

Table 1. Ways to decrease homologous transfusions.

- Eliminate transfusion "triggers"
- Increase use of autologous transfusions
  - preoperative donations
  - perioperative hemodilution
- intraoperative salvage
- intervene pharmacologically
  - control of hemostasis
  - recombinant growth factors
- expand bone marrow/stem cell transplantation

It is likely that implementing the alternative strategies that prove cost effective will result in profound changes in blood centres as they move toward the next century.

As an aside, although the public concerns and this essay focus on the infectious disease risks of transfusion, the potential immunosuppressive effects of red cell transfusions provide an additional impetus to reduce transfusion exposures. These adverse effects have been known for some time [5]. Although a consensus has not developed about their seriousness or frequency, many surgeons are sufficiently concerned about immunosuppression effects to seek transfusion alternatives for their patients to avoid the risks. Detailed prospective studies will be required before the risks are defined and appropriate practices developed [6].

Blood transfusion avoidance

Strategies to avoid the transfusion of homologous blood are outlined in Table 1. Some of these strategies are evolving, while others are becoming established Transfusion Practice.

Transfusion "triggers"

Transfusion "triggers" described by Friedman and associates [7] refer to laboratory or clinical values that result in decisions to transfuse. Many of these thresholds, such as 10 g per dl of hemoglobin as a trigger for red cell transfusions, are supported by scant scientific data. Thus, patients are now released from hospitals with less than 8 g of hemoglobin per dl. Levine and associates reported that chronic anemia (hemotocrit, 15%) had no apparent adverse affect on baboons [8]. In an accompanying editorial, Stehling and Zauder question whether these findings can be safely extrapolated to man [9]. They further point out that safe levels of anemia will be more accurately defined in man based on data derived from increasingly widespread use of physiologic monitoring in various clinical settings. Whatever level of anemia may ultimately be determined to be safe, the demise of transfusion triggers, at least for red cells, is imminent. The commonly used transfusion trigger of 20,000 platelets per μl may be more stubborn. However, in place of triggers, transfusion therapy will be tailored to the clinical needs of specific patients. Noting that a specific safe level of hemoglobin does not exist, experts on blood transfusion of the Council of Europe recently emphasized that transfusion therapy must be individualized [10].

Autologous transfusions

Autologous transfusion issues were recently reviewed extensively [11] and guidelines were also recently published by the Council of Europe [12]. It is clear that preoperative autologous donations remain underutilized [13,14], but it is unclear why this is so. It has been demonstrated that autologous transfusion referrals by surgeons correlate with their understanding of autologous practice: The better the understanding, the more appropriate use of autologous transfusions [15]. Thus, intensified educational efforts may improve use of autologous transfusions. The recent report that recombinant human erythropoietin (rhEPO) increases the tolerance of patients to preoperative phlebotomy [16] may increase further both the scope and safety of preoperative donations for autologous use.

Supplementing oxygen delivery during perioperative hemodilution with acellular oxygen-carrying solutions is an exciting second form of autologous Transfusion Practice [11,17]. Formulations of both hemoglobin and perfluorocarbons currently advocated as "blood substitutes" have insufficient intravascular dwell time to serve as true substitutes for blood. However, they may be suitable to augment oxygen delivery in patients who would be unlikely to tolerate reduced oxygen-carrying capacity during perioperative hemodilution or are unable to donate enough blood prior to surgery to meet their transfusion needs. Early trials with a perfluorocarbon emulsion in animal models suggest this approach may be successful [18,19]. Without regard to whether oxygen can be supplemented, increased use of perioperative hemodilution offers an excellent opportunity to reduce homologous blood use in the future.

The use of intraoperative salvage of shed blood in the operating room, a third form of autologous transfusion, was recently reviewed extensively by Williamson and Taswell [20]. As further data become available about its safe use in patients with malignancy and infection, intraoperative salvage can take its place beside preoperative donation as standard practice [20].

Pharmacologic management of hemostasis and anemia

Desmopressin (DDAVP) has been used in various hemostatic conditions, especially platelet function disorders and von Willebrand's disease, to shorten the bleeding time during and following surgery [21]. However, the data from open heart surgery in patients with normal hemostasis is not in agreement. Salzman and associates found DDAVP reduced perioperative blood loss associated with open heart surgery [22], but Hackmann and associates could not confirm the efficacy of DDAVP in this setting [23]. The use of aprotinin also continues to be reported as valuable in reducing the need for red cell transfusions during several types of surgical procedures [24]. Use of these drugs will continue to be explored as interventions to reduce red cell and platelet transfusions.

As noted, rhEPO increases the tolerance to autologous donations and thus can reduce homologous needs. The efficacy of rhEPO in end-stage renal disease has dramatically reduced the red cell transfusion needs of these patients [25] and in other forms of chronic anemia as well [26]. Early trials in the administration of rhEPO in a variety of other clinical settings, such as prematurity and in the perioperative period, are underway [27]. *Preliminary analysis of ongoing trials of rhEPO in the perioperative period indicates reduced exposure to homologous blood in patients undergoing coronary artery bypass surgery* [Adamson J, personal communication, 1991]. Other recombinant human growth factors may prove to have many applications in Transfusion Medicine [28]. The use of GM-CSF in aplastic anemia has been beneficial [29]. More recently, GM-CSF enhanced neutrophil recovery and promoted early engraftment following autologous bone marrow transplantation [30]. These applications of growth factors clearly have the potential to avoid homologous transfusions and their use is likely to be expanded.

Bone marrow transplantation

The prospect that chronic anemias, both acquired and hereditary, may respond to bone marrow or stem cell transplantation is offering hope to patients previously doomed. Many of the lifelong anemias require frequent blood transfusion, especially of red cells. Alloimmunization and hypersiderosis are common complications, in addition to the constant risk of acquiring infectious diseases. The success of transplantation in children with severe thalassemia is especially encouraging. In one study, 75% of 222 patients were event-free at one year following transplantation of fully compatible homologous marrow [31]. Bone marrow transplantation of HLA haploidentical partially matched donors has also been reported to result in 28% event-free survival in patients with thalassemia [32]. Early success has been achieved in related marrow transplants in two sickle disease patients in Cincinnati [Harris R, personal communication, 1991]. Marrow transplantation in aplastic anemia has also been beneficial [33,34] and stem cell transplantation for Fanconi's anemia using umbilical cells has shown limited efficacy [35]. Since most patients with Fanconi's anemia do not survive past 20 years of age, this is yet a further exciting transfusion alternative that also increases survival. For each of these expanding roles for hematopoietic cell transplantation, the requirements for lifelong homologous transfusion support will decrease.

Process and quality engineering of blood centres

As screening blood donors and the testing and processing of donated blood has grown increasingly complex, so has the opportunity for manufacturing errors, whether clerical or technical. In 1981, blood centres performed two tests to prevent disease transmission by transfusions, hepatitis B surface antigen and syphilis. Ten years later, eight tests are performed to protect transfusion recipients from acquiring infectious diseases from their transfusions. This proliferation of tests and the resulting data have increased, pari passu, the opportunity for clerical and computer errors, either of which may result in the release of components unsuitable for transfusion. The problems these complex systems pose have been illustrated in the United States by deficiencies in blood centre operations found during inspections by the Food and Drug Administration (FDA). Process and management inadequacies continue to be the principal cause of acute deaths from transfusions [36]. Although there is no clear evidence that any of the findings on the 483s (standard FDA form used to cite establishment deficiencies found during an inspection) issued to blood centres by the FDA resulted in transmission of disease to recipients, the findings do suggest that improved quality and process engineering must be undertaken, at least in centres in the United States.

Blood centres traditionally have been held to standards of performance outlined in the 600 Series of the Title 21, Code of Federal Regulations (CFR). But, as political pressures to improve the safety of the blood supply intensified in the United States, the FDA began to apply the more stringent 200 Series. The elements of good manufacturing practices (GMP) – especially Section 211 – have been stressed. Analysis of inspectional findings by the FDA offers the opportunity not only to address the findings, but, more importantly, to institute changes in GMP that permitted the findings to occur. The key elements of GMP are listed in Table 2.

Compliance with GMP will be enhanced by introducing process and quality engineering into blood centres. In industrial quality science, the recognition, analysis, and elimination of variation is a fundamental principle [37]. But, these principles have been underemphasized in health care organizations [37]. The traditional static modes of quality assurance that focus on outcome analysis have been overtaken in industrial settings by analysis of variation. This new focus recognizes that complex interactions dictate development of new methods for quality control.

Table 2. Elements of good manufacturing practices (GMP).

- Record keeping
- Validation
- Calibration
- Error management
- Personnel training
- Process/production controls
- Quality assurance/self-audit
- Facility and equipment maintenance
- SOPs/written procedures

Table 3. Elements of effective error management.

- Error/incident reporting
- Error/incident analysis
- Corrective action
- Validation of corrective action

Organizations must undertake continuous improvement in their quality [38]. Successful continuous improvement must become a cultural phenomenon within an organization – instinctive compliance with GMP must become embedded in an organization's culture. Although the medical profession in general has been slow to embrace models of continuous improvement, blood centres can take a leadership role in these efforts.

Not only has the FDA become concerned about quality engineering in health care, but also the Joint Commission on Accreditation of Health care Organizations (JCAHO) which, through inspections, sets health care inpatient standards in the United States. The JCAHO has established task forces to determine suitable quality indicators for all major medical specialties [39]. Increasing emphasis in process and quality can be felt during JCAHO inspections, especially in Transfusion Medicine settings.

Reduction in lot-to-lot variations is one of the principle objectives of the GMP provisions of Title 2 – that the establishment consistently releases products that are of high quality and conform to the provisions of its license. In the context of blood centres, insuring that the components released for transfusion have been appropriately processed and tested, especially for evidence of viral contamination, is the objective of GMP.

Reduction of lot-to-lot variation has two key elements: Error management and personnel training. The elements of error management are outlined in Table 3. As noted, continuous improvement concepts must be embedded in the culture of an establishment and error recognition and reporting by the staff is an important aspect of this culture. The process is known to the Japanese as poka-yoke or "mistake proofing" [40]. This process assumes that production employees will have lapses that result in defects or errors. Rather than focusing on the outcomes of such lapses or the person who had the lapse, poka-yoke focuses on the systems or processes that permitted the error to occur. Further, employees are encouraged to report errors and are not punished for experiencing lapses. To draw from the Japanese again, the spirit is embodied in their epigram, "Every defect is a treasure" [38]. Every employee in a blood centre can be empowered to stop a process with which they have found a problem that could result in the release of components unsuitable for transfusion.

The second element of error management is analysis. Once an error has occurred, the designs of the systems and processes that permitted the error to effect outcome are meticulously reviewed. The cause or causes may not be immediately obvious, but the analysis continues until the design flaw is found.

Corrective action forms the third element of error management and is at the heart of both process engineering and the theory of continuous improvement. Instituting appropriate process and system design changes to prevent error recurrence results in overall quality improvement. Error analysis may reveal that employees are not adequately trained for the tasks they perform. This is not an employee problem, but more frequently the result of inadequate training – a systems failure.

Finally, any process or system design change must be validated by determining whether the design changes did what they were expected to do. Some "improvements" may affect other parts of a system in such a way that matters are actually made worse. This is especially true when computer systems have been modified. thus, it is important to validate the entire system in which changes are made.

Duplicate donor records universally pose problems for blood centres and how this weakness was approached by our centre illustrates the four elements of error management. When we failed to disqualify a unit from a repeat donor who was on the donor deferral registry for a repeatably reactive HIV-1 enzyme-linked immunoassay (EIA), it was clear we had a design flaw in our data management. First, the error was reported to the FDA. Second, error analysis instructed us that two errors had been made at the second donation, one by the donor who changed his social security number slightly, and one by the records clerk who made an error in entering the donor's name. As a result, when the donor donated the second time, the record of his prior, and disqualifying, donation could not be matched by the computer. A new – duplicate – record was created and it did not match the data in the deferral registry.

The corrective action to prevent similar errors in the future involved designing and installing a computer program, which was the third step in error management. Entitled "DUPE", this program matches donor record number and letter strings seeking possible duplicate pairs and flags any units that could be from a donor with similar data strings; that is, come from a donor who had a duplicate record. The program was installed as part of donor processing and was validated. A unit must clear this DUPE program before it can be labelled. Approximately 7 in 300 donor records contain data that requires further analysis to assure that a duplicate record has not been created for a person already on the donor deferral registry [41].

The second key aspect of the reduction in lot-to-lot variation is personnel training. Major pharmaceutical companies *may devote up to 60 hours per year in training experienced manufacturing personnel* and maintain even more extensive training programs for new personnel [Cagliotti T, Johnson and Johnson, personal communication, 1991]. These companies have learned that intensive training of personnel is critical to reduce errors. Blood centres, at least in the United States, generally have not invested in training as intensively as the pharmaceutical industry. Yet, as blood centres are held to higher standards of performance that is of equal rigor to that of the pharmaceutical industry, such training programs will be required [Cardin M, FDA National Expert, CCBC Meeting, Des Moines, IOWA, July 1991].

Table 4. Elements of effective personnel training.

- Hands-on didactic and technical training
- Certification
- Documentation

Table 5. Strategies to remove/inactivate viruses.

- Heating
- Filtering
- Washing
- Treating with solvent-detergents
- Photoinactivating
- Treating with lasers
- Combination treatment

Effective training programs have three key elements (Table 4). Hands-on didactic and technical training are provided to insure that the technical personnel understand the standard operating procedures filed, at least for United States license holders, with the FDA. At our centre, additional personnel are being hired in the viral testing laboratory to permit an "annual training sabbatical" to be taken by each employee in the section. During this period their main focus is retraining and it is their principal duty. In the United States much publicity has been given to the American National Red Cross's plan to close all activities in about 10% of its centres in rotation to permit "transformation". During closure the staff would be intensively trained in uniform operating procedures.

The second element of training is certification, the analog of validation for systems. In our centre, following retraining, the nursing staff take a certification examination to test their knowledge of the nursing operating procedures. Personnel who fail are given additional training.

Finally, documentation of both the training and certification are essential to meet both regulatory requirements and to assure that the centre is meeting the professional standard of care. Documentation should be in both the employees' personnel files and in the quality control records of the centre. Extensive training and certification programs are expensive. The Red Cross has estimated that its transformation process will cost over 120 million dollars for its 52 centres [42]. However, the costs of such programs have been recovered in the pharmaceutical industry through fewer product recalls and increased productivity.

Viral inactivation of blood components

Because improving donor screening and testing and introducing continuous improvement practices in blood centres will only reduce but not eliminate release of unsuitable units for transfusion, viral inactivation is viewed by many to be the next plateau of transfusion safety. In part, this view is held because of the transfusion transmitted diseases we do not know about – ten years ago we were unaware of HIV-1. Many different inactivation strategies have been proposed and were recently reviewed [43]. However, some workers appear pessimistic about overcoming the many problems posed by viral inactivation [44]. Some of the probable strategies to inactivate or remove viruses are outlined in Table 5.

Two very different problems are presented to developers of viral inactivation of blood components. The first is to inactivate commercial fractions, plasma components, principally fresh-frozen plasma and cryoprecipitate, that is, the acellular infusions. The second is to process fresh cells, principally red cells and platelets, in a manner to inactivate both viable viruses and intact proviruses.

Inactivation of acellular products and components

Several technologies are available to inactivate viruses in fractionated commercial products and fresh or fresh-frozen components. The earliest inactivation efforts used heat to destroy the as yet unidentified non-A, non-B agent, now referred to as hepatitis C (HCV) in clotting factor concentrates [45]. Epstein and Frike recently reviewed progress in this area [46]. Although *in vitro* studies indicated a high degree of efficiency in eliminating viruses with dry heat [47], dry heated factor VIII commercial concentrates, although not dry-heated factor IX concentrates, have been shown to transmit HIV-1 [48]. Even though pasteurization has been shown to inactivate hepatitis viruses in factorVIII concentrates [49], commercial companies have turned to more harsh treatments. In the United States, most commercial fractions are inactivated by solvent detergent treatment [50,51]. This process, using tri-butyl phosphate and sodium cholate, has been shown to be effective in inactivating both viral hepatitis agents as well as HIV-1 [50]. In Europe, other techniques, including inactivating plasma with beta-propriolactone [52] and steam have been used [53].

Inactivation technology is being applied developmentally to fresh or fresh-frozen as well as commercially fractionated products. Successful solvent-detergent treatment of a fibrin glue preparation has been reported [54].

Inactivation of cellular components

Inactivating viruses in cellular components poses much more difficult challenges than in acellular components. As noted, many agents act by destroying the lipid envelopes of the viruses. These same agents are destructive of the membranes of both platelets and red cells. This may prevent the use of the more harsh solvents and detergents in cellular component systems.

Second, several viruses of interest, especially the retroviruses, are partitioned, at least in part, within white cells. Further, their genetic material integrates as provirus into the genome of the host cell. Some, such as cytomegalovirus and HTLV-I/II, are exclusively partitioned within white cells. Although this may serve as an advantage in that white cell removal will be effective, it is unlikely that all leukocytes can be removed. High-efficiency filters were developed to prevent alloimmunization by white cells and buffy-coat reactions, but their use to remove intracellular viruses is of increasing interest. Further, filtration technology is improving rapidly and reductions of white cells to less than 10^5 per red cell unit are possible [55,56]. It is becoming evident that removal to this level will, in and of itself, reduce the transfusion risk of cytomegalovirus [57], although other viruses, such as HIV and HCV, may behave differently. It is also clear that although cellular debris is removed, infectious particles are still found in the remaining fluid [58]. A cautionary note has been sounded recently. Leukocyte removal has been found to reduce the bacteriocidal properties of blood drawn for transfusion [59]. In an accompanying editorial, Heal urges caution and suggests that it is too early to tell whether white cell removal is good or bad [60].

The partitioning of the various viruses and the integration of some into white cells may require multiple strategies to be combined to successfully inactivate viruses in cellular components. At the current state of development, it appears that filtration of white cells and chemical/photoinactivation treatment will be combined.

Psoralens

In the psoralen family, aminomethyltrimethylpsoralen (AMT) and 8-methoxypsoralen (8-MOP) plus UV light have been reported to inactivate HBV and non-A, non-B agents in plasma [61]. Platelet concentrates have also undergone viral inactivation by treating them with 8-MOP and long wavelength UV light [62]. When this family of compounds is excited by UV light, they fuse complementary strands of nucleic acids and unstranding for replication is prevented. Thus, provirus as well as free virus could be inactivated, provided the compounds can bind to the nucleic acids of intact white cells. Because of its action on nucleic acids, concerns have been raised about whether they would induce mutagenicity from altered DNA.

Porphoryrins

Among the porphyrins, benzoporphyrin derivative (BPD) exposed to red light has been shown to inactivate marker viruses in blood [63] and a dihematoporphyrin ether (DHE) has been shown to be virucidal for HIV-1 as well [64]. It is not completely understood how porphyrins and visible light inactivate viruses, but is believed to be related to both their lipophilic properties and the formation of toxic oxygen singlets when excited by light. A porphyrin-like compound, aluminum phthalocyanine, has also been found to inactivate both cell-associated and cell-free vesicular stomatitis virus (VSV) in red cell suspensions [65].

Dyes

Several dyes have been found to inactivate viruses when excited by visible light. Among these are the phenothiazine dyes, methylene blue and toluidine blue [66], and merocyanine 540 (MC 540) [67]. As noted the porphyrin-like dye, aluminum phthalocyanine, inactivates viruses. Each has been shown to be effective in inactivating both cell-associated and cell-free viruses in suspensions of red cells. Although these compounds are lipophilic and also bind to nucleic acids [66], the viral inactivation mechanism is unclear.

Other

Although it is beyond the scope of this essay to discuss all compounds proposed to inactivate viruses, some are of special interest. The methods described above require visible or UV light to excite the inactivating compound. This may be difficult to achieve in systems that are practical. Among other chemicals proposed that do not require light, hypericin is reported to inactivate both DNA and RNA viruses, but requires a lipid envelope to be effective [68]. Hypericin has been used as an antidepressant in man and tolerance could be anticipated, perhaps without requiring removal prior to transfusion. Caprylate is a second agent that is effective against enveloped viruses [69]. Caprylate would require removal either by complexing or washing of the cells. Neither of these compounds require excitation by light.

Concerns have been raised about any of the chemical or photochemical strategies proposed [44]. The first is the residual dose of the proposed photo-inactivating agents even after removal. Although the dose may be acceptable for single units, the massively transfused patient and the exchanged transfused neonate may be exposed excessively. Extensive studies in models must address this problem.

Second, studies reported to date have used crude methods to evaluate red cell or platelet membrane damage. Because many of the candidates are lipophilic, cell membranes may be equally attractive as virions. It would seem that detailed analysis of membrane effects are critical early in the evaluation of a strategy. Most of the studies published have used crude measures, such as hemoglobin release from red cells, to determine cellular integrity. More sophisticated cellular studies are needed and early ones reported reinforce concerns about damaged cell membrane lipid [70].

One of the most attractive inactivation methods is the use of pulsed lasers to inactivate DNA and RNA at wavelinks that highly excite nucleic acids, but spare proteins and lipids. Laser light has been shown to be effective in inactivating marker viruses in platelet concentrates [71]. This technology is especially attractive because no "additive" is required and toxicity from residual agents would not be of concern. Further, most of the chemical inactivation strategies are only effective against enveloped viruses. Nonenveloped viruses are transmitted by transfusions, most notably parvoviruses, the causative agents of fifth disease [72]. Other nonenveloped viruses transmitted by transfusions are likely to emerge in the future. Thus, although delivery of the appropriate dose of laser light may require elaborate processing equipment that would be difficult to scale-up, direct DNA and RNA inactivation of blood components would be an important development.

Because it would solve so many problems facing blood centres today, it is clear that much research and further development in viral inactivation will be undertaken in this decade. And I believe that successful systems be developed. It is probable that combinations of strategies will be needed. Whether the cost of the technology is proportionate to the risk will await the unfolding of the new methodology.

Summary

In this essay I have attempted to identify future trends in Transfusion Medicine. Because current strategies for protecting the safety of blood transfusions have reached practical limits, I have focused on alternatives to transfusion of homologous components as a continuing endeavour. Further, I believe that methods to improve the quality and process controls of the collection, processing and distribution systems currently in place will undergo major improvements that will effect not only the designs of the systems themselves, but also our culture. The impact on our culture has already been felt. The changes are affecting us not only as a profession, but as we go about our daily lives in our centres. Last, intense efforts will be focused on virus-inactivating cellular components. This may be the most difficult task of all. But, we will pursue it in order to remove the greatest fear the public has about receiving a transfusion – succumbing to AIDS.

References

1. Zuck TF, Greetings – a final look back with comments about a policy of a zero-risk blood supply (editorial). Transfusion 1987;27:447-8.
2. Cumming PD, Wallace EL, Schoor JB, Dodd RY. Exposure of patients to human immunodeficiency virus through the transfusion of blood components that test antibody-negative. N Engl J Med 1989;321:941-6
3. Busch MP, Elbe BE, Khayam-Bashi H, et al. Evaluation of screened blood donations for human immunodeficiency virus type 1 infection by culture and DNA amplification of pooled cells. N Engl J Med 1991;325:1-5.
4. Mayo DJ, Rose AM, Matchett SE, Hoppe PA, Solomon JM, McCurdy KK. Screening potential blood donors at risk for human immunodeficiency virus. Transfusion 1991;31:466-73.
5. Fischer E, Lenhard V, Siefert P, Kluge A, Johannsen R. Blood transfusion-induced suppression of cellular immunity in man. Hum Immunol 1980;3:187-94.
6. Alexander JW. Transfusion-induced immunomodulation and infection (editorial). Transfusion 1991;31:195-6.
7. Friedman BA, Burns TL, Schork MA. An analysis of blood transfusion of surgical patients by sex: A quest for the transfusion trigger. Transfusion 1980;20:179-88.
8. Levine E, Rosen A, Sehgal L, Gould S, Sehgal H, Moss G. Physiologic effects of actue anemia: Implications for a reduced transfusion trigger. Transfusion 1990; 30:11-4.

9.Stehling L, Zauder HL. How low can we go? Is there a way to know? (editorial) Transfusion 1990;30:1-2.

10.Gunson HH. Transfusion: News from the Council of Europe. Committee of Experts on Blood Transfusion and Immunohaematology: Abridged report of 1st meeting held in Liège in May 1989. Vox Sang 1990;58:324-7.

11.Zuck TF, Carey PM. Autologous transfusion practice. Controversies about current fashions and real needs. Vox Sang 1990;58:234-42.

12.Council of Europe. Guidelines for autologous blood transfusion. A consensus opinion of the Committee of Experts on Blood Transfusion and Immunohematology. Vox Sang 1989;57:278-80.

13.Toy PTCY, Strauss RG, Stehling LC, et al. Predeposited autologous blood for elective surgery. N Engl J Med 1987;316:517-20.

14.Popovsky MA, Wells HJ, Page PL. Autologous transfusion: Evidence of continued underutilization (abstract). International Society of Blood Transfusion/American Association of Blood Banks Joint Congress, Los Angeles, 1990. Abstract S506, p.127.

15.Strauss RG, Ferguson KJ, Stone GG, et al. Surgeons' knowledge, attitude and use of preoperative autologous blood donations. Transfusion 1990;30:418-20.

16.Goodnough LT, Rudnick S, Price TH, et al. Increased preoperative collection of autologous blood with recombinant human erythropoietin therapy. N Engl J Med 1989;321:1163-8.

17.Messmer K, Kreimeier U, Intaglietta M. Present state of intentional hemodilution. Eur Surg Res 1986;18:254-63.

18.Hogan MC, Willford DC, Wagner PD. Effect of perfluorooctobromide emulsion on O_2 diffusing capacity of dog muscle working maximally in situ with low [Hb] (abstract). Biomaterials, Artificial Cells, and Immobilization Biotechnology 1991;19:398

19.Braun RD, Goldstick TK, Linsenmeier RA. Concentrated perfluorooctylbromide emulsion infusion increases tissues PO_2 in normovolemic cats breathing 100% oxygen (abstract). Biomaterials, Artificial Cells, and Immunobilization Technology 1991;19:360.

20.Williamson KR Taswell HF. Intraoperative blood salvage: A review. Transfusion 1991;31:662-75.

21.Schulman S. DDAVP – the multipotent drug in patients with coagulopathies. Transfusion Med Rev 1991;5:132-44.

22.Salzman EW, Weinstein MJ, Weintraub RM, et al. Treatment with desmopressin acetate to reduce blood loss after cardiac surgery: A double-blind randomized trial. N Engl J Med 1986;314:1402-6.

23.Hackman T, Gascoyne RD, Naiman SC, et al. A trial of desmopressin (1-desamino-8-D-arginine vasopressin) to reduce blood loss in uncomplicated cardiac surgery. N Engl J Med 1989;321:1437-43.

24.Royston D, Bidstrup BP, Taylor KM, Sapsford RN. Effect of aprotinin on need for blood transfusion after repeat open-heart surgery. Lancet 1987;ii:1289-91.

25.Eschback JW, Egrie JC, Downing MR, Browne JK, Adamson JW. Correction of the anemia of end-stage renal disease with recombinant human erythropoietin. N Engl J Med 1987;316:73-8.

26.Bunn FH. Recombinant erythropoietin therapy in cancer patients (editorial). J Clin Oncology 1990;8:949-50.

27.Erslev AJ. Erythropoietin. N Engl J Med 1991;324:1339-44

28.Groopman JE, Molina J-M, Scadden DT. Hematopoietic growth factors. N Engl J Med 1989;321:1449-56.

29.Vadhan-Raj S, Buescher S, Broxmeyer HE, et al. Stimulation of myelopoiesis in patients with aplastic anemia by recombinant human granulocyte-macrophage colony-stimulating factor. N Engl J Med 1988;319:1628-34.

30. Lazarus HN, Anderson J, Chen MG, et al. Recombinant granulocyte-macrophage colony-stimulating factor after autologous bone marrow transplantation for relapsed non-Hodgkins's lymphoma: Blood and bone marrow progenitor growth studies. Blood 1991;78:830-7.

31. Lucarelli G, Galimberti M, Polchi P, et al. Bone marrow transplantation in patients with thalassemia. N Engl J Med 1990;322:417-21.

32. Galimberti M, Lucarelli G, Polchi P, et al. HLA-mismatched bone marrow transplantation in thalassemia. Bone Marrow Transplantation 1991;7(supp.3):98-100.

33. Storb R, Chamblin RE. Bone marrow transplantation for severe aplastic anemia. Bone Marrow Transplantation 1991;8:69-72.

34. Socie G, Gluckman E, Devergie A, Girinsky T, Esperou H, Cosset JM. Bone marrow tranplantation (BMT) for acquired severe aplastic anaemia (SAA): Long term follow-up of 107 consecutive patients (abstract). Bone Marrow Transplantation 1991;7(supp.2):102.

35. Broxmeyer HE, Kurtzberg J, Gluckman E, et al. Umbilical cord blood hematopoietic stem and repopulating cells in human clinical transplantation. Blood Cells 1991;17:313-29.

36. Sazama K. Reports of 355 transfusion-associated deaths: 1976 through 1985. Transfusion 1990;30:583-90.

37. Laffel G, Blumenthal D. The case for using industrial quality management science in health care organizations. JAMA 1989;262:2869-73.

38. Berwick DM. Continuous improvement as an ideal in healh care. N Engl J Med 1989;320:53-6.

39. Labovitz GH. The total-quality health care revolution. Quality Progress 1991; Sept:45-7.

40. Shengo S. Zero quality control: Source inspection and the poka-yoke system. Cambridge, MA. Productivity Press, 1986.

41. Simpson LE, Zuck TF. Detecting duplicate donor computer records in spite of differences in key fields (abstract). Transfusion 1991;31(supp.):838.

42. Hilt PJ. Red Cross Orders Sweeping Changes at Blood Centers. New York Times. 10 May 1991:1(1).

43. Wagner JS, Friedman LI, Dodd RY. Approaches to the reduction of viral infectivity in cellular blood components and single donor plasma. Transfusion Med Rev 1991;5:18-32.

44. Frantantoni JC, Prodouz KN, Horowitz MS. Viral inactivation of blood products (editorial). Transfusion 1990;30:480-1.

45. Hollinger FB, Dolana G, Thomas W, Gyorkey F. Reduction in risk of hepatitis transmission by heat-treatment of human factor VIII concentrates. J Infect Dis 1984; 150:250-62.

46. Epstein JS. Fricke WA. Current safety of clotting factor concentrates. Arch Pathol Lab Med 1990;114:335-40.

47. McDougal JS, Martin LS, Cort SP, Mozen M, Heldebrant CM, Evatt BL. Thermal inactivation of the acquired immunodeficiency syndrome virus, human T-lymphotropic virus-III/lymphadenopathy-associated virus, with special reference to anti-hemophilic factor. J Clin Invest 1985;76:875-7.

48. Dietrich SL, Mosley JW, Lusher JM, et al. Transmission of human immunodeficiency virus type 1 by dry-heated clotting factor concentrates. Vox Sang 1990; 59:129-35.

49. Schimpf K, Mannucci PM, Kreutz W, et al. Absence of hepatitis after treatment with a pasteurized factor VIII concentrate in patients with hemophilia and no previous transfusions. N Engl J Med 1987;316:918-22.

50. Prince AM, Horowitz B, Brotman B. Sterilisation of hepatitis and HTLV-III viruses by exposure to tri(n-butyl)phosphate and sodium cholate. Lancet 1986;i: 706-10.

51. Horowitz B, Wiebe ME, Lippin A, Stryker MH. Inactivation of viruses in labile blood derivatives. I. Disruption of lipid-enveloped viruses by tri(n-butyl)phosphate detergent combinations. Transfusion 1985;25:516-22.

52. Hoppe I. Hepatitis safety of a new prothrombin complex preparation, sterilized according to the methods of LoGrippo. Blut 1985;50:363-8.

53. Wober G, Dorner F, Eibl H, et al. Steam treatment of freeze-dried plasma fractions (abstract). Hemostasis 1985;15:13.

54. Burnouf-Radosevich M, Burnouf T, Huart JJ. Biochemical and physical properties of a solvent-detergent-treated fibrin glue. Vox Sang 1990;58:77-84.

55. Reverberi R, Menini C. Clinical efficacy of five filters specific for leukocyte removal. Vox Sang 1990;58:188-91.

56. Freedman J, Blanchette V, Hornstein A, et al. White cell depletion of red cell and pooled random-donor platelet concentrates by filtration and residual lymphocyte subset analysis. Transfusion 1991;31:433-40.

57. Bowden RA, Slichter SJ, Sayers MH, Mori M, Cays MJ, Meyers JD. Use of leukocyte-depleted platelets and cytomegalovirus-seronegative red blood cells for prevention of primary cytomegalovirus infection after marrow transplant. Blood 1991;68:246-50.

58. Rawal B, Yen TSB, Vyas GN, Busch M. Leukocyte filtration removes infectious particulate debris but not free virus derived from experimentally lysed HIV-infected cells. Vox Sang 1991;60:214-8.

59. Högman CF, Gong J, Eriksson L, Hambraeus A, Johansson CS. White cells protect donor blood against bacterial contamination. Transfusion 1991;31:620-6.

60. Heal JM. Do white cells in stored blood components reduce the likelihood of post-transfusion bacterial sepsis? (editorial) Transfusion 1991;31:581-3.

61. Alter HJ, Creagan RP, Morel PA, et al. Photochemical decontamination of blood components containing hepatitis B and non-A,non-B virus. Lancet 1988;ii:1446-50.

62. Lin L, Wiesehahn GP, Morel PA, Corash L. Use of 8-methoxypsoralen and long-wave-length ultraviolet radiation for decontamination of platelet concentrates. Blood 1989;74:517-25.

63. Neyndorff HC, Bartel DL, Tufaro F, Levy JG. Development of a model to demonstrate photosensitizer-mediated viral inactivation in blood. Transfusion 1990;30:485-90.

64. Mathews JL, Sogandares-Bernal F, Judy MM, et al. Preliminary studies of photo-inactivation of a human immunodeficiency virus in blood. Transfusion 1991;31:636-40.

65. Horowitz B, Williams B, Rywkin S, et al. Inactivation of viruses in blood with aluminum phthalocyanine derivatives. Transfusion 1991;31:102-7.

66. Lambrecht B, Mohr H, Knuver-Hopf J, Schmitt H. Photoinactivation of viruses in human fresh plasma by phenothiazine dyes in combination with visible light. Vox Sang 1991;60:207-13.

67. Sieber F, Krueger GL, O'Brien JM, Schober SL, Sensenbrenner LL, Sharkis SJ. Inactivation of friend erythroleukemia virus-transformed cells by merocyanine 640-mediated photosensitization. Blood 1989;73:345-50.

68. Tang J, Colacino JM, Larsen SH, Spitzer W. Virucidal activity of hypericin against enveloped and non-enveloped DNA and RNA viruses. Antiviral Research 1990;13:313-26.

69. Lundblad JL, Seng RL. Inactivation of lipid-enveloped viruses in proteins by caprylate. Vox Sang 1991;60:75-81.

70. Koerner IAW, Walker KE, Strauss RG, Lin L, Piete W, Wiesehahn G. Effect of 8-methoxypsoralen and UVA irradiation on the composition of platelet and lymphocyte lipids (abstract). International Society of Blood Transfusion/American Association of Blood Banks Joint Congress. Los Angeles, 1990, Abstract S489,p.123.

71. Prodouz KN, Fratantoni JC, Boone EJ, Bonner RF. Use of laser-UV for inactivation of viruses in blood products. Blood 1987;70:589-92.
72. Williams MD, Cohen BJ, Beddal AC, Pasi KJ, Mortimer PP, Hill FGH. Transmission of human parvovirus B19 by coagulation factor concentrates. Vox Sang 1990;58: 177-81.

AN IMPROVEMENT IN THE SUPPLY OF SAFE BLOOD: VIRUS INACTIVATED PLASMA PREPARED IN THE BLOOD BANK

Y. Piquet[1], G. Janvier[2], P. Selosse[3], E. Angevain[1], J. Jouneau[1], G. Nicolle[1], C. Doutremepuich[4], G. Vezon[1]

To reduce virus infectivity in blood products, several methods were attempted. Selection and then screening of volunteer donors (HBsAg, anti-HIV Ab, anti-HBc Ab, anti-HCV Ab, ALAT) have reduced the likelihood of viral transmission. Despite all the screening tests and the purification methods used to produce therapeutic stable protein solutions, the best method for further reducing viral risks is the introduction of a viral inactivation step in the procedure. For albumin, pasteurization [1] on the final product has been found to be an effective way for viral sterilization and until now no case of hepatitis B has been attributed to pasteurized albumin. For coagulation factors, the first method used was the heating of concentrates in the lyophilised state [2] to kill HIV virus. Improvement has been achieved by including a solvent detergent method in the procedure to inactivate all viruses [3].

Unfortunately, for labile derivates, it is still not possible to inactivate viruses, except in fresh frozen plasma. In 1987, Horowitz [4] has reported that the inactivation of plasma is possible, and recently a technique using a solvent detergent method has been developed.

Thus, in order to eliminate the possible transmission of viruses by plasma, we decided to apply this method in our blood bank. Several batches were prepared to check biological parameters, the recovery of coagulation factors and their possible activation.

1. Centre Régional de Transfusion Sanguine, place Amlie Raba-Lon BP 24, 33035 Bordeaux Cedex.
2. CHU Pellegrin 33000 Bordeaux.
3. Octapharma A.G., Schweizerohtstrasse 1, 8750 Glarus, Switzerland.
4. Facult de Pharmacie de Bordeaux, Rue Leyteire, 33000 Bordeaux.

Material and method

Virus inactivation of plasma

For virus inactivation, we used a procedure licensed by Octapharma Laboratories. Batches were composed of two categories of plasma: Plasma collected by automated plasmapheresis and plasma recovered from whole blood donations.

Plasma bags were frozen at –40°C immediately after plasmapheresis or within six hours after whole blood collection. Six lots with a mean volume of 60 litres were prepared. After thawing in a thermostated tank, plasma was filtered through 1 μm porous filters into an other tank placed in a clean room (class 10,000). Virus sterilization was performed by incubating plasma with 1% (w/w), TnBP and 1% (w/w) Octoxynol 9 for four hours at 30°C. Following the virucidal treatment solvent detergent reagents were removed from proteins, using castor oil and chromatographic treatment on insolubilized C18. After chromatography, the pH of plasma was adjusted to 7.4 and the plastic bags were aseptically filled to a volume of 200-220 ml. Then, the bags of plasma were frozen to –40°C and stored at –30°C.

Biological parameters

Coagulation factors

Factor VIIIC, IX, XI and XII activity was measured by a one step method [5] based on the activated partial thromboplastin time using reagents supplied by Diagnostica STAGO. The factor VIIIC content was calculated using a national standard provided by the French "Laboratoire National de la Santé".

The reference used for factors XII, XI and IX was a pooled citrated plasma from 30 healthy individuals. Normal coagulation factors values are considered to be at 1 U/ml.

Factors II, V, VII and X were assayed using the prothrombin time method [6] with deficient plasma (Diagnostica STAGO) and a pooled citrated plasma as reference.

AT III activity was measured by an amidolytic assay (AT Prest STAGO) [7], and von Willebrand factor activity using platelet aggregation in the presence of the plasma to be studied and of ristocetin [8]. Fibrinogen levels were determined by a previously described method [9].

Activated factors

Factor IXa activity was measured using the method described by Vinazzer [10] whose principle is based on the fact that factor IXa molecules are fixed on AT III. An amidolytic method was used to measure the activity of factor Xa [11]. The non-activated partial thromboplastin test was carried out according to the method described by Kingdon et al. [12] for factor IX concentrates. Plasma was tested with no dilution. In vivo thrombogenicity was determined using the Wessler method [13].

Biochemical parameters

Total protein content was measured by the Biuret method [14], free hemo-globin using tetramethyl benzidine [15], sodium and potassium by flame photometry, and osmolarity using an osmometer. Endotoxin levels were per-formed using a chromogenic assay [16]. The assay of Octoxynol 9 was de-veloped by Octapharma Laboratories; 5 ml of the plasma solution were passed through a C18 resin and packed in a chromatographic column. Standards should be treated in the same manner. After washing with distilled water, iso-propanol was used for elution of a fraction containing Octoxynol 9. The eluate was then concentrated to approximatively 0.2 ml. Distilled water was added to bring the volume to 1 ml. Samples were chromatographed on a 3.9 mn 30 cm column (Waters) with an HPLC analyser. A linear gradient with distilled water and isopropanol was employed and Octoxynol 9 was detected at 230 nm with a UV detector. Typical chromatographs were obtained and Octoxynol 9 quantified by comparing the area of the peak with that of standards.

TnBP was assayed by gas chromatography using a Delsi apparatus equipped with a 10% SP 1000 column. 3 ml of sample were placed in a 15 ml centrifuge tube, containing 2.5 g of sodium sulfate. 10 µl of TNPP were used as an internal standard. 1 ml of ethanol and 1 ml of perchloric acid were added and brought to 37°C for 10 minutes. After vigorous mixing, 4 ml of hexane were added and the sample was then centrifuged. The organic phase was re-covered and evaporated. Each sample was diluted in 30 µl of hexane. 0.3 µl were injected in the chromatograph. Oven temperature was 170°C and nitrogen flow rate was 30 ml/mn. Chromatographic peaks were recorded and compared to standards (3 µg/ml, 5 µg/ml and 10 µg/ml) which were assayed under the same conditions as the sample to be tested.

Results

Coagulation factors

The mean level of coagulation factors II, V, VII, IX, XI, XII were all over 0.7 IU/ml (Table 1). Because there are no available concentrates for factor V and XI deficiency, it is important to note that levels found in virus inactivated plasma were respectively 0.78 IU/ml and 0.85 IU/ml.

After the chromatographic stage, a small dilution occurred and 92% of total initial protein was recovered. So, the recovery of coagulation factors was al-most total (Table 2). Only values of factor VIII, a labile parameter, decreased and the recovery from initial plasma was 73.76%. It is important to note that in our table we do include the first batch prepared. Factor V is less sensitive than factor VIII to virus inactivation. All tests on the activation of coagulation factors were negative (Table 3). The times obtained with the NAPPT test are all over 150 s. Values for Xa factor determination are within the normal range. The values found for activated factor IX fall within the standard deviation of the assay of factor IX.

Biochemical parameters are mentioned in Table 4. Mean protein level is

Table 1. Levels of coagulation factors in virus inactivated plasma.

Lots	II U/ml	VII U/ml	IX U/ml	X U/ml	XI U/ml	XII U/ml	VIIIC U/ml	V U/ml	vWF U/ml	AT III U/ml	FIB g/l
PVI 1	0.96	1	0.93	0.95	0.79	1.04	0.54	0.73	1.1	0.75	2.53
PVI 2	0.92	1	0.85	0.75	0.95	0.95	0.7	0.9	1.05	1.05	2.12
PVI 3	0.93		0.9	0.9	0.75	1.1	0.86	0.95	1.05	0.96	2.03
PVI 4	0.88	1.05	0.95	0.88	0.78	1.15	0.67	0.82	1.1	0.86	1.83
PVI 5	0.82	0.95	0.72	0.8	0.7	1.1	0.7	0.88	0.7	0.98	2.01
PVI 6	0.88	1.05	0.72	0.9	0.72	1.15	0.65	0.9	0.8	1.12	2.18
Mean	0.89	1	0.84	0.86	0.78	1.08	0.68	0.85	0.96	0.95	2.11
SD	0.04	0.03	0.1	0.07	0.08	0.07	0.1	0.08	0.17	0.13	0.23

Table 2. Recovery (%) of coagulation factors after viral inactivation of plasma. (Protein recovery = 91.92%)

Factor	PVI 1	PVI 2	PVI 3	PVI 4	PVI 5	PVI 6	Mean %	SD
Factor II	99	92	93	93.6	80.39	89.7	91.2	6.15
Factor VII	100	100	100	100	91	96.33	97.88	3.68
Factor IX	93	85	90	90	79.12	77.41	85.75	6.36
Factor X	95	87	94.7	97.7	77.66	90	90.34	7.3
Factor XI	98.7	100	77.3	91.7	87.5	92.3	91.25	8.27
Factor XII	100	86.3	100	95.8	95.65	100	96.29	5.32
Factor VIIIC	67.5	75	83.49	78.82	68.63	69.15	73.76	6.45
Factor V	85.8	100	86.36	79.82	81.48	90	87.2	7.27
von Willebrand factor	100	93.7	95.4	88	82.35	88.88	73.76	6.24
AT-III	93.7	96.3	99.5	81	91.58	98.24	93.38	6.72
FIB	83.3	100	96	90	92.2	93.97	92.57	5.68

Table 3. Activated factors in virus inactivated plasma.

Lots	NAPTT	IXa %	Xa U/ml	Wessler test
PVI 1	> 150 s	2	0.046	negative
PVI 2	> 150 s	3.4	0.041	negative
PVI 3	> 150 s	0	0.046	negative
PVI 4	> 150 s	3	0.043	negative

54.71 g/l, sodium 155.9 mmol/l and potassium level is lower than 5 mmol/l. The levels of TnBP and Octoxynol 9 are below the detection limit of methods. The endotoxin level is 0.83 EU/ml which is not very high. These values are confirmed by the pyrogen test being negative.

Discussion

Virus inactivated plasma meets the legal requirements for French frozen plasma specifications concerning protein (50 g/l) and potassium levels (< 5 mmol/l). The specifications also require at least 0.7 IU/ml of factor VIIIC and 0.7 IU/ml of factor V. We have proved in our study that factor V level is not significantly affected by virus inactivation. The decrease of factor VIII level is more significant. Thus in processing plasma intended for viral sterilization care must be taken to preserve maximum levels of labile coagulation factors. Several factors can induce a loss of factor VIIIC. Firstly, the process itself must be as short as possible. From the thawing of plasma, the procedure takes fifteen hours. Secondly, the techniques by which plasma is collected vary and it is well known that plasma obtained by plasmapheresis contains higher levels of factor VIIIC than plasma from whole blood donation [17]. It is also important to establish with the other blood centres, good plasma freezing and storage practices [18].

Several authors have studied other methods for improving the viral safety of plasma. It was proved that laser UV irradiation [19] with exposure doses between 10.8 and 21 j/m2 inactivates viruses. The plasma prothrombin time and activated partial thromboplastin time are used as general indicators of laser UV treatment on plasma coagulation factors. These two parameters, as opposed to the values with our procedure, are higher with irradiated plasma samples. Nevertheless with this procedure it is difficult to extrapolate what proteins are affected.

Other workers [20] have used photoactivated dyes for virus inactivation of blood and have described a decrease of fibrinogen levels in plasma. Hamamoto et al. [21] propose a filtration method with hollow fiber membranes. HIV viruses are fixed due to the multilayer structure of the filter. Trials have also been performed for the inactivation of the immunodeficiency virus by gamma radiation [22]. The authors have shown that to recover 85% of coagulation

Table 4. Biochemical parameters of virus inactivated plasma.

Lots	pH	Total protein g/l	Free hemoglobin mg/l	Sodium mmol/l	Potassium mmol/l	Osmolarity mosmol/l	Endotoxins EU/ml	TnBP µg/l	Octoxynol µg/l
PVI 1	7.41	56.5	56	126.9	3.33	316	0.69	< 1	< 5
PVI 2	7.49	54.7	51	150	3.22	–	0.77	< 1	< 5
PVI 3	7.55	56.1	61	162.6	3.32	318	0.74	< 1	< 5
PVI 4	7.54	52.6	69	150.2	3.06	287	1.52	< 1	< 5
PVI 5	7.45	52.8	83	150.9	3.22	313	0.67	< 1	< 5
PVI 6	7.53	56.47	85	158.8	3.41	334	0.61	< 1	< 5
Mean	7.48	54.78	67.83	155.9	3.26	313.6	0.83	< 1	< 5
SD	0.058	1.72	14.56	6.23	0.12	16.94	0.34		

factors, the irradiation doses cannot exceed 1.4 MRad which is an inadequate dose for the inactivation of HIV virus. Because of the presence of the endogenous lipid of plasma, unsaturated fatty acids are not convenient for virus inactivation [23]. The solvent detergent method seems to be the best method, both because it has proved its efficacy on viruses and also the good recovery of coagulation factors [24]. In a recent report [25] Horowitz indicates the absence of neo-antigens and a good recovery of coagulation factors. In all these published works nobody has done assays on activated factors. We think this is necessary to prevent thrombosis in patients receiving virus inactivated plasma. In our work, some activated factors were studied. All of them were negative. The absence of factor IX will probably be confirmed in future batches in NAPTT, which is sensitive to this factor, was found to be negative.

Based on these laboratory studies and with the aim of improving the supply of safe products, fresh frozen plasma can be replaced by virus inactivated plasma.

References

1. Gellis S, Neefe J, Strong l, Janeway C, Scatchard G. Chemical, clinical and immunological studies on products of human plasma fractionation: Inactivation of virus of homologous serum albumin by means of heat. J Clin Invest 1948;27:239-44.
2. Hollinger JB, Dolano G, Thomas W, Gyorkey F. Reduction risk of hepatitis transmission by heat treatment of a human factor VIII concentrate. J Inf Dis 1984;150: 250-64.
3. Horowitz B, Wiebe ME, Lippin A, Stryker MH. Inactivation of virus in labile blood derivates. I. Disruption of lipid-enveloped virus by tri/n/buthyl/phosphate detergent combinations. Transfusion 1985;25:216-9.
4. Horowitz B. Virus sterilization of plasma protein by treatment with solvent detergent mixtures. A summary. Thromb Res 1987;48(supp.VII):51 (abstract).
5. Biggs R, Evelin S, Richards G. The assay of anti-haemophilic globulin activity. Br J Haemat 1955;1:20-34.
6. Soulier JP, Larrieu MS. Etude analytique des temps de Quick allongés. Dosage de prothrombine, de proconvertine et de pro-accélérine. Sang 1982;23:549-59.
7. Odegard OR, Lie M, Abilgaard U. Heparin cofactor activity measured with an amidolytic method. Thromb Res 1975;6:287-94.
8. Howard MA, Firkin BG. Ristocetin: A new tool in the investigation of platelet aggregation. Thromb Diath Haemorrh 1971;26:362-9.
9. Clauss A. Gerinnungs physiologische Schnellmethode 2 in Bestimmung des Fibrinogens. Acta Haemat 1975;17:237-46.
10. Vinazzer H. Comparison between two concentrates with factor VIII inhibitor bypassing activity. Thromb Res 1982;26:21-9.
11. Martinoli JL, Doussin G, Nigham F. Automatisation de l'étude de l'hémostase et de la fibrinolyse par les substrats chromogéniques. Nouv Rev Franç Hématol 1981; 23(supp.):L (abstract Proc. VIe CSFG, Avignon).
12. Kingdon HS, Lundblad ML, Veltkamp JJ, Amonson DL. Potentially thrombogenic materials in factor IX concentrates. Thromb Diath Haemorrh 1975;33:617-31.
13. Wessler S, Reiner S, Sheps MC. Biological assay of a thrombosis inducing activity in human serum. J Appl Phys 1959;14:943-53.
14. Gornall A, Bardawill CH, David M. Determination of serum protein by means of the biuret reaction. J Biol Chem 1949;177:751-66.

15.Elson EC, Ivor L, Gochman N. Substitution of a non hazardous chromogen for benzidine in the measurement of plasma haemoglobin. Am J Clin Path 1978;69: 354.
16.Thomas LLM, Sturck A, Kahle LH, ten Cate JW. Quantitative endotoxin determination in blood with a chromogenic substrate. Clin Chem 1981;116:63-8.
17.International Forum. What are the critical factors in the production and quality control of frozen plasma intended for direct transfusion or for fractionation to provide medically needed labile coagulation factors? Vox Sang 1983;44:246-59.
18.Carlebjork G, Blombäck M, Pihlstedt P. Freezing of plasma and recovery of factor VIII. Transfusion 1986;26/2:159-62
19.Prodouz KN, Fratantoni JC, Boone EJ, Booner RF. Use of laser UV for inactivation of virus in blood products. Blood 1987;70:589-92.
20.Mathews JL, Newman JT, Sogandares-Bernal F, et al. Photodynamic therapy of viral contaminants with potential for blood banking application. Transfusion 1988; 28:80-3.
21.Yoshiaki H, Shinsi H, Sumunu K, et al. A novel method for removal of human immunodeficiency virus: Filtration with porous polymeric membranes. Vox Sang 1989;56:230-6.
22.Hiemstra H, Tersmette M, Vos H, Over J, van Berkel MP, Debree H. Inactivation of human immunodeficiency virus by gamma radiation and its effect on plasma and coagulation factors. Transfusion 1991;31:32-9.
23.Horowitz B, Piet PJ, Prince AM, Edwards CA, Lippin A, Walakovits ML. Inactivation of lipid enveloped viruses in labile blood derivates by unsaturted fatty acids. Vox Sang 1988;54:14-20.
24.Piet MPJ, Chin S, Prince AM, Brotman B, Cundell AM, Horowitz B. The use of tri-n-butyl phosphate detergent mixtures to inactivate hepatitis viruses and human immunodeficiency virus in plasma and plasma's subsequent fractionation. Transfusion 1990;30:591-8.
25.Horowitz B, Chin S, Prince AM, Brotman B, Pascual D, Williams B. Preparation and characterization of S/D-FFP, a virus sterilized "fresh frozen plasma". Thromb Haem 1991;65:1163 (abstract).

TRANSFUSION MEDICINE TODAY AND TOMORROW: THE FACTS AND THE FICTIONS

J.D. Cash

In the early 1970s the World Health Organization became increasingly concerned at the long-term prospects for the safety and availability of blood and blood products. So much so that it subsequently called for countries to develop national blood transfusion services which were committed to self-sufficiency and acquired their blood from unpaid donors. Few countries took a serious interest in these recommendations, although significant progress was made in some countries to support the concept of the unpaid donor.

In 1978 the Council of Europe's Expert Committee on Blood Transfusion and Immunohaematology was restructured and reorganized and there began a series of important in-depth studies of Transfusion Practice throughout Europe, which continue to this day and which have in the last decade had an increasingly important impact throughout Europe and beyond. By the early 1980s sufficient data had been collected to reveal that there were significant problems in the provision of blood transfusion support for health care programs throughout Europe. The Expert Committee concluded that one of the major deficiencies was a paucity of high quality professional leadership.

The Expert Committee sought to explore ways of resolving some of these difficulties and it concluded that energies should be directed towards the education and training needs of staff in major regional (community) blood centres. In this context the Committee reaffirmed previous deliberations that all directors of such centres should be medically qualified. Against these backgrounds a Working Party was established by the Expert Committee to bring forward proposals for the education and training of medical doctors who wished to work (full time) in major regional (community) blood centres. I was privileged to be a member of this Working Party.

The Working Party brought forward its proposals in 1984. They were approved by its parent Expert Committee and in 1985 received the approval of the Council of Ministers [1]. The fundamental new position which emerged from these extensive consultations and deliberations was the creation of a prospect – an opportunity – for the emergence of a new medical specialty which in some countries is now called Transfusion Medicine. These European centred activities have been viewed with much interest in other parts of the world, notably Japan and Australasia. In North America, particularly the USA, Transfusion Medicine has also emerged, although it seems probable that its origins and roots may be somewhat different: Emerging out of the conflagration of AIDS and rooted primarily in high quality research and undergraduate and postgraduate teaching to future and existing key prescribers of blood and blood products.

The recent issue of the EEC Directive (Directive 89/381) [2] in which many of those original 1975 WHO exhortations will become espoused within the European political movement is a major new development and has inevitably given rise to a desire to re-analyze the place and relevance of Transfusion Medicine in Europe, against the background of a political initiative to develop programs designed to achieve national and Community self-sufficiency in high quality blood products. In the 1990s particular emphasis in this political initiative has been put upon quality assurance and good manufacturing practice and we should note that the Council of Europe's Expert Committee already had foreseen this development [3]. The EEC Directive has also stressed, as did its WHO originator, the notion that an integral part of self-sufficiency must be considerations not only of supply but of demand – prescribing preferences and practices. The European politicians have also called for appropriate attention to be given, in any plans directed towards Community self-sufficiency, to the emergence of biotechnology derived blood related products.

It comes as no surprise that in due course an initiator of this second look at Transfusion Medicine might emanate from the northern part of the Netherlands, that the nature of the Groningen challenge would be characteristically vigorous and tinged with scepticism. Some would suggest that the motion before the house in this Groningen debate should be "that Transfusion Medicine is a fiction". How different from the attitudes of colleagues from southern Europe, who will seek to encourage discussions in Prague[1] designed to explore the adaptations required in the 1990s for the implementation of proposals developed by the Council of Europe in the early 1980s.

Yet these differences are more apparent than real, for in a sense they both seek to address, at least in part, an undeniable fact: There has, since Ministers approved on the Expert Committee's proposals in 1985, with the exception of the United Kingdom, been relatively little response. One must conclude that in some way the medicine prescribed by the European Expert Committee in 1984 was inappropriate: Perhaps too rich an admixture of facts and fictions and of dreams and realities.

Blood Transfusion Practice is that total activity which links the blood donor to the patient. There are three distinct operational supports to this bridge:
– the blood collection process;
– donation testing and processing; and
– the clinical interface.

1. 3rd Regional Congress, European Region of the ISBT, october 1991.

We should not forget that successful Transfusion Practice is dependent on many other skills that are made available from professionals other than medical practitioners and perhaps in the future the Expert Committee of the Council of Europe will give consideration to the training of these groups. Nonetheless it follows that Transfusion Medicine can best be described as those functions within this bridging exercise which it is believed should be undertaken by medical practitioners.

There can be little doubt that the vision the Council of Europe's Expert Committee had of Transfusion Medicine was based upon an operational circumstance which can best be described as the complete bridging process. Thus it was considered that a practitioner of Transfusion Medicine would contribute to the blood collection, donation testing and processing and the clinical interface. Accordingly, the proposed education and training programs sought to ensure that the qualified medical practitioner was able to practice effectively in all these areas, including management practice.

Looking across Europe we must conclude that there are very few blood centres in which this vision of Transfusion Medicine is a reality. Many are dominated by blood collection and donation processing and testing and have no operational locus at the clinical interface. Others, claiming to practice Transfusion Medicine, acquire their blood supplies from external sources and direct all their professional energies to the clinical interface. The nature of this clinical interface can vary substantially between different institutions; there are some in which the medical practitioners are familiar, because they are actively involved each day, with the clinical use of all blood components and plasma derivatives and are frequently to be seen in the clinical environments. In other institutions plasma derivatives are not acquired by clinicians through the hospital blood bank but from the hospital pharmacy, and in many such institutions the primary tool used by the Transfusion Medicine specialist is the telephone.

For those who look for fictions, then the prescriptive approach of the Council of Europe to the definition or the boundaries of Transfusion Medicine may find some support. They would argue that it is not based on operational reality and that until this is realized, the newly created specialty cannot and will not flourish. They will point to the way general surgery and internal medicine in the last 20 years have separated into a series of sub-specialities and that the reverse process – the bringing together of separate parts, each with high levels of knowledge, is a phenomenon that runs counter to reality in the latter part of the twentieth century, particularly when some of those parts are already firmly based in other medical sub-specialties and as such are jealously guarded.

It is an interesting fact that over the past two days our hosts, supported by many excellent individual speakers, have provided us with a feast of the separate constituents which make up much of what at least the European founding fathers believed were the bases of Transfusion Medicine. There can be no doubt that the admixture is exhilarating and challenging but its operational reality varies from country to country and often within any one country.

As we look to the future it seems to me that at least in Europe we will see the inexorable development of Transfusion Practice and the speciality of Transfusion Medicine, primarily because blood transfusion has become of interest to politicians, but also because of expanding patient need and public demand. Slowly but surely some of the fictions will become facts as politicians wrestle with the extraordinary demands of this remarkable European initiative – self-sufficiency based on the unpaid donor. It seems certain that one of the key elements in this development will be the establishment of academic centres of excellence that are primarily concerned with new product developments, prescribing practice and safety. The endeavours of the Council of Europe in the 1980s are to be applauded but should be seen as the first round in a continuing debate. It is time for the next generation of medical practitioners to sit down and deliberate on future strategies. There seems little doubt that this occasion in Groningen can be viewed as a watershed and that in the second debate the morality and ethics of blood Transfusion Practice will come to the fore and in doing so will disrupt many of the principles upon which Transfusion Practice has hitherto been based. We may well see the diminution in influence of the hospital pharmacist in movement of plasma products towards the bedside and the politicians begin to realize that the voluntary unpaid donor principle is not well suited to marketplace forces.

But perhaps the major future debate for those who seek to ensure that Transfusion Practice (and thus Transfusion Medicine) is the total activity from donor to patient, will be resolving the fundamental conflict of interest of those who seek to supply (the more the better) and those who seek, at the clinical interface, to curb the prescription of blood and blood products on the grounds of safety and cost benefit. The politicians are now involved in blood Transfusion Practice in Europe and as a consequence Transfusion Medicine will flourish.

The Council of Europe's Expert Committee has played a critical role in catalyzing much that is good in Transfusion Practice in Europe. Perhaps the single message that should emerge from this 16th Groningen Symposium on Blood Transfusion is that we should use what influence we have to persuade the Expert Committee to have another look at Transfusion Medicine. It would seem clear that further refinements and evolution are necessary.

References

1. Council of Europe. Study of the current position of training programmes for future specialists in blood transfusion in Council of Europe member states and in Finland. ISBN 92-871-0757-2.
2. EEC Directive 89/381/EEC.
3. Council of Europe. Report on quality control in blood transfusion services. Strassbourg 1986. ISBN 92-871-0851-X.

DISCUSSION

U. Rossi, C.Th. Smit Sibinga

D. Goldfinger: We heard over and over again, that blood transfusion is safe. We keep hearing this as though as we keep saying it, it is really to become true. It cannot be stated this way. In the future when we find ways of inactivating viruses in cellular components then perhaps we can make this statement, but today we cannot. We said it was safe in the eighties, because we were making great headway with the control of transfusion associated hepatitis. But along came a disease we had never heard of, or never even imagined. Today while testing for many diseases we can only say that perhaps it is safer. However, since we have a one out of 4000 chances to get HIV, even this is debatable. We certainly cannot say that it is safe regarding diseases that we have never heard of, or that we have heard of but do not know of being transmitted by blood transfusion.

The second point is the statement that the safest transfusion is the one not given. I think that is too, a jargon among blood bankers; we used to call ourselves blood bankers before we called ourselves Transfusion Medicine specialists. I think all too often blood bankers were viewed as if they were like regular bankers; once they got the blood in their blood bank, they did not want to give it out. It is true that there is many an unnecessary transfusion and it is better that that transfusion is not to be given. But when a patient really needs a transfusion then it is not a true statement that the safest transfusion is the one not given, since the patient is likely to die for lack of a transfusion. So, I think we have to stop talking to our clinical colleagues as though they are idiots, as though they always transfused incorrectly and that they need this paternalistic kind of an approach to withhold transfusion. I think at times that is a useful approach, but all too often it is not. There is another role for us at the clinical side. How often do we see the blood banker actually recommending an additional transfusion? We do it at our own place the whole time. I think that there are many times that transfusions are given unnecessarily, but there is a place for us in the clinical management of critically ill patients where withholding transfusions or talking to the clinican is though as he is giving too much, is not necessarily in our best interest or in the patient's.

C.Th. Smit Sibinga: I think it is very true what Dr. Goldfinger is saying. There is the dogma on the one hand, but there is the bridge aspect on the other hand. We are coming to where these two sides of the bridge reach each other: The clinical consultative responsibility.

T.F. Zuck: The first information presented, was in the context of public perception. I agree with you, we know the viruses probable transmitted and we do not have a test for them. We know that transfusions are not completely safe, but the information was set up in context of public opinion. I agree with you we must say it is not safe, but it is much safer, in fact, than the public perception. In terms of a transfusion not given, I suppose you could add unnecessary transfusion, but you can not say, in my view, that a transfusion not given does not transmit disease.

C.F. Högman: I would just refer to Dr. P. Lundsgaard-Hansen who always advocated moderation in this similar thoughts as Dr. Goldfinger expressed, namely that the problems for the clinician to know when a transfusion is really important. Then quite recently he referred to some work indicating that in fact silent ischaemia without any symptoms is much more common than has been known before and this I think would underline caution in going too far in not transfusing patients.

J.D. Cash: Those of us who have been in Transfusion Medicine for many years know that a lot of patients have received blood when they really did not need it. We have much difficulty in addressing this problem because we still have insufficient methods to define an individual patient's "transfusion trigger". In this context I am particularly interested in some new instruments, that may tell us levels of tissue oxygen which in turn indicate the need for red cell transfusions. Thus at the present time we honestly have great difficulty with the level of our precision in prescribing which seems greater than in many other areas of medicine. It is my hope that these problems will be tackled in the next decade and I think the SANGUIS Group in leading us in the right direction.[1]

H.J. ten Duis (Groningen, NL): Well as a clinician I think that we must be aware of the fact that every transfusion be it plasma or red cells, is potentially dangerous. In my opinion in five or ten years it will not be necessary anymore to transfuse plasma in surgical patients. If we are looking at our practice in trauma-surgery at this moment, a healthy young trauma patient who goes down with the hematocrit value and hemoglobin to 6 g/l should not be given any blood transfusion before some signs of ischemia on the ECG appear. When that is not the case we do not transfuse the healthy young patient. We allow a hematocrit down to about 20% and even lower in the Jehovah's witnesses.

1. Ten Duis HJ, McClelland DBL, p. 169–76.

That leads to extension of the hospitalisation time, but they will survive at a very low hematocrit.

D.B.L. McClelland: I would like to make three points really to the discussion. First, when talking about transfusion management of a patient we should avoid making generalizations of a kind that we would think were bizarre, if we were talking about any other kind of management of the patient. It is the job of a clinician to look at a patient as an individual and use the knowledge and experience in his specialty to tailor and look for treatment for the patient. So, I completely agree with a blood transfusion trigger that would be different but appropriate for transfusion treatment of individual persons.

Second, it would be extremely interesting and very important for us to have access to powerful mechanisms of looking at the clinical physiology associated with for example red cell transfusion. We should remember that red cells are a long standing therapeutic product, but as far as I know never has been subject to clinical trials to establish indications and dosage. Access to new devices might allow us to see in the patient more accurately what happens when you transfuse red cells. However, we should not forget that the main point that we have to look at is the end-result for the patient. What the patient is interested in is three things: Number one survival; number two feeling well and number three getting out of the hospital and getting back to work. There are amazingly few studies that I am aware of relating to either Transfusion Practice, the use or non-use of autologous transfusion or any other aspect of what we do, that have actually looked at the patient outcome.

The final comment I would like to make is drawn from an observation made by Dr. Heather Hume who has done some beautiful work in pediatric transfusion audit in Canada.[1] It is borne out very strongly by the SANGUIS study and which shows that one of the first steps to improving practice in transfusion would be to insist that clinicians write in the patients' case records the reason why an individual transfusion was ordered. That was only done in about 30% of the case records reviewed in the SANGUIS study. I believe that one of the first ways of improving individual medical practice is to insist that people write down and sign for the reasons they did what they did.

F. Peetoom: I guess this is the last chance to verify perceptions that I have developed over the last two days. It looks to me that the European Transfusion Community has a different set of priorities at this time than the one that we are exposed to in the United States. In this session, we have seen again the manufacturing side as well as an attempt to identify what the role is of a transfusion practitioner. They are obviously complementary, possibly synergistic. However, in the United States we certainly focus on somewhat different areas.

1. Hume H. Paediatric transfusion: Quality assessment and assurance. In: Sadner RA, Strauss R (eds). Contemporary issues in paediatric transfusion medicine. American Association of Blood Bankds, Arlington VA. 1989:55-80.

Maybe that is good, because after all we are a world community and we probably should combine our interests and come up with solutions that will be useful to each other. The differences in priorities are not incompatible, just different aspects of a broad field of issues, and these are all important. Now, I have a question though: I think the political agenda in the United States is pretty clear. We have a Congress with its oversight committees directing the FDA. As a result, the focus on blood product manufacturing is a clear consequence of a political agenda. We hear about the EEC having a political agenda. In Europe the politicians are also becoming involved. But it is not clear to me what the operational implications are of such involvement. I do not think that the politicians are involved with the identity crisis of transfusionists, and they probably have something else in mind. I would like someone to tell me what are the operational implications of the political interests at the EEC level.

J.D. Cash: The major difference between the United States of America and Europe is that there is a movement developing in Europe, generated by politicians who are saying this: We have in the past relied upon commercial companies to supply us with large amounts of plasma pooled products, fractionated products. When we look at this, the major source of companies' plasma supply is from paid donors. It would appear from those of us in Europe that it comes as no surprise that it is so, because the industry developed. But in Europe they decided we wish now to move down a track – it is the politician speaking – in which the source of product is ultimately stopped and that the community looks after itself and it does that from the base of the unpaid donor. The impact of that decision affected series of organizations that have relied traditionally for two, three decades on a major input coming from the commercial sector of North America, the paid donor to be told we are moving into an era, in which we have to stand on our own. The impact of that and we are standing on our own dominantly from recovered plasma in the first instance, has a major impact on these transfusion services. Many of them established traditionally in the fifties, the sixties and the seventies in this context have been fast asleep. To them it is a major cultural shock and inevitably that is going to have an impact as it evolves on the people that are working in these services.

F. Peetoom: We have heard about the European plasma self-sufficiency plan for some time. I had the impression that there might be more to the political agenda than just the plasma issue. Of course, this plan has many years of work left to be done.

J.D. Cash: Although the concept of European self-sufficiency will prove a difficult one to deliver, I believe it will be achieved in Western Europe sooner than many contemplate.

B. Habibi: First of all I would like to sincerely thank the speakers of this symposium, all of them, for their very stimulating and thoughtful contributions.

Then I would like to make four brief comments.

First, I think, two important statements were made by Dr. Goldfinger and Dr. Zuck. Dr. Goldfinger's statement was: "The clinicians are not idiots" and Dr. Zuck quoting Dr. Bovie's statement that the best transfusion is the one not given. I am a bit puzzled by those two statements. I think that clinicians are not idiots; transfusion people at the other side of the bridge are not idiots either. I just think that all of us dramatically need clinical scientific data. That is the main problem. Why do we observe such wide variations in use as reflected in the SANGUIS project. That is something that we are observing for decades in Europe and the United States. Why? Because the area is difficult. Clinical investigation in Transfusion Medicine is one of the most difficult areas to be dealt with. We have to promote such kind of investigation.

Second, the interaction of politicians in this medical area and the fact that they show more and more interest in Transfusion Medicine is actually a revolutionary aspect we are witnessing. One of our main tasks these days, is to devote a substantial amount of our energy in informing them and communicating with them. They should have been, and they will be an integral part of Transfusion Medicine over the next decade. What would be useful in my mind is to promote also the idea of the quality assurance in legislative and regulatory actions and procedures. This should be put into action and promoted in one way or another.

The third brief remark relates to Dr. Piquet's communication regarding the inactivation of whole plasma. I think that is a very important achievement with two main advantages. The first, obvious for all of us is providing a safer product to the patient, but the other I think still more important is to reduce the use of fresh frozen plasma, because of the high cost of the new product, to its real indications, if that product has any real clinical indication.

The last remark will be focused on the ethics of blood donation and transfusion. I think during these very stimulating two-and-a-half days we have not enough focused on the issue of ethics, but mainly on the safety of non-remunerated blood donations. Blood cannot be sold, it cannot be the subject of any profit: This is one of the fundamental aspects of Transfusion Medicine that I perceive as a fact even if in 1991 it seems to be partially still a fiction.

B.T. Teague: A couple of comments and a question. The first comment relates to the safe versus unsafe issue. I think AIDS could be renamed the "oops" disease in terms of blood banking. Many blood bankers said things, that turned out to be absolutely false although they were said in good conscience based on current data, i.e. blood was safe as it related to AIDS; this was before it was determined that it was transmissible. However, I think we will be reminded for these things for a long time to come. But the good news of that is that today many people are much more sensible about what they say and they are much more careful to be able to document what they say. It is best not to put your mouth in motion until you put your brain in gear. I think a lot of people are learning that over with the AIDS issue.

Second, in terms of usage, inappropriate usage, I believe there is substantial data and I applaud the SANGUIS project. I think that would be great to do in our own region, which has 109 facilities, but I believe the shortage segments around the world have also proven that there is inappropriate use in many areas. It is amazing to see physicians get along with less than they usually do in shortage times and still the patients do very well. We should take that as a lesson. Sometimes the availability has to go down before appropriate use can be done. I do not mean that in a general term, but I think there are selected cases and those should be looked at.

The third item plus the question is, that this has been an ever stimulating symposium. We talk about what is different in Europe and the US of North America and there are differences. But it is also abundantly clear that the world has shrunk, communication has improved and we must do a better job of working together as a world entity. So that one group can learn from the errors or the experiences of others and prevent those same things happening in another part of the world. In the terms of ethics and administration I think there is so much to be learned. But my question is how do we merge these two continents, how do we set up the bridge so that we bring all the players onto it and get cooperation and education from all the sources in order to make everyone a little better provider.

C.Th. Smit Sibinga: I will take up that question and wind up the meeting together. I think what we have heard and learned over these days stand against a perspective which Dr. Hu gave in his introductory presentation. We are again focusing on the developed part of the world, the highly industrialized part of the world, the part of the world that struggles with the problems: How can we reduce usage, how can we increase safety, what measures can we take, politicians coming in, Council of Europe etc. I am not even talking about the implications of the lawyer's system in the United States; we have heard the concept of the voluntary non-remunerated lawyer to be introduced in our field. The point is the tremendous increase in speed of developments. It goes that fast that actually today and tomorrow, there will already have been instituted changes, which are far away from the majority of this world which is still in the stages of the first generation blood transfusion organization and even less than that, where focus has been on some technical aspects, like blood grouping and cross-matching, but all the other aspects have been out of the scope. There should be an awareness more on the making of mistakes and errors, we should indeed treasure each error we find and try to get to a better understanding and implementation of qualities of education in our centres. If we start doing that from both the sides of the bridge, I think we will get somewhere. That actually brings me to what Dr. Klein just said on the future developments, the implementation specifically of biotechnology. It is very fascinating although that is the spearhead of the developments. Coming down to reality, I think we should try to recognize also that the major risk today in blood transfusion is not in the infections and is not even in the restrictions so much as was put forward as a concept, but is in the paucity and lack of education on a structured, integrated basis in Transfusion Medicine spreading from the one side of the bridge to the other side. A second point is the non-acceptance, as it still is, of Transfusion Practice into the entire mainstream of clinical medicine. These are two fundamental things. We start recognizing that and start to implement them and bring them into practice both in the developing countries as well as in the industrialized world. I think we might get somewhere over the next decade. I would refer to a recommendation from a recent consultation at WHO in Geneva[1] defining Transfusion Medicine: *Transfusion Medicine deals with that part of the health care system, which undertakes the appropriate provision and use of human blood and blood resources* and the concept of the bridging process to which a medical practitioner could contribute, which holds in its essence also the contributions of many, many other disciplines within the field of health care, including pharmacy.

I think we should wind up the meeting with these thoughts, which might balance the facts and the fictions a little better. Thank the speakers warmly for their contributions.

1. Informal consultation WHO/GBSI, Geneva 23-26 September 1991.

INDEX

DEVELOPMENTS IN HEMATOLOGY AND IMMUNOLOGY

DEVELOPMENTS IN HEMATOLOGY AND IMMUNOLOGY

KLUWER ACADEMIC PUBLISHERS – DORDRECHT / BOSTON / LONDON